Bump & Grind

The A–Z survival guide
for when you're trying to get pregnant
and sick of being told to *relax!*

Genevieve Morton
Illustrated by Fiona Katauskas

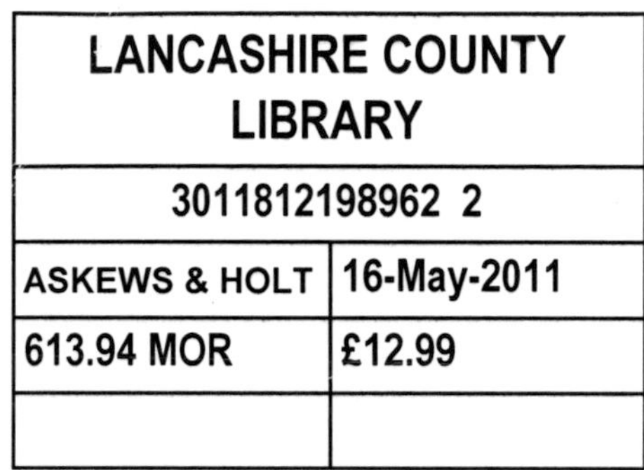

Bump & Grind: The A–Z survival guide for when you're trying to get pregnant and sick of being told to relax!

Important note:

The information in this book is not intended as a substitute for medical advice. Neither the author nor White ladder Press can accept any responsibility for any injuries, damages or losses suffered as a result of following the information herein.

This first edition published in 2011 by White Ladder Press, an imprint of Crimson Publishing, Westminster House, Kew Road, Richmond, Surrey TW9 2ND.

Originally published in 2010 in Australia and New Zealand as *Bump & Grind: The A–Z survival guide for when you're trying to get pregnant and sick of being told to relax!* by Finch Publishing Pty Limited, Sydney, Australia.

British Library Cataloguing in Publication Data

A catalogue record for this book is available from the British Library.

ISBN 978 1 90541 088 0

Typeset by IDSUK (DataConnection) Ltd.

Printed and bound in the UK by Ashford Colour Press, Gosport, Hants.

CONTENTS

CONTENTS

INTRODUCTION

Nobody say 'relax!'

If one more person said 'Just relax and you'll get pregnant!' when I was trying to have a baby I would have torn out an ovary just to have something to chuck at them. There is nothing relaxing about Trying To Conceive (TTC) when you have spent months and months upside down riding an imaginary bike or scissor-kicking the ceiling. Somewhere between 'Maybe I'm not ovulating' and 'Maybe you're not aiming it right' you realise TTC just isn't fair. Some women – I call them Smug Fertility Goddesses (SMGs) – seem to get pregnant after sniffing their husband's dirty socks, and then go on to brag about it. Others get pregnant after a few well-timed trysts on holiday. The rest of us have to work at it, and do I mean *work*. Along with charting our temperature, observing our cervical mucus and nagging our partners about their tight undies and fourth beer, there is the emotional roller-coaster of TTC which no book I've read can prepare you for. Like when the latest Smug Fertility Goddess at work announces she's pregnant (again!) on the day you get your period (again!) and you spend the morning crying in the office bathroom. Or when a male colleague asks you when you're going to 'squeeze out a few puppies' because you're not getting any younger – the week after your fourth failed round of IVF. Or, when a caring but clueless aunt informs you the only way to get pregnant is to stop *worrying* dear because in her day, they 'didn't even think about it!'

TTC is hard, *hard* work. And it's often lonely work. Most of us don't share our TTC efforts with the world because we don't want to jinx our luck, we fear failure, or because we just couldn't stand it if one more person nudged us with 'So, how's it going? Anything yet?' as if we are waiting for the arrival of the baby we bought on eBay. We join online chat forums to vent our frustrations and share our deepest fears. We soldier on, month after month, waiting for a positive pregnancy test. We cry, we pray, we try to get healthier, and we hope our partner will eventually understand why we threw out his high-cut bikini briefs …

My own TTC story goes like this …

My husband Ben and I started trying for a baby when I was 34 years old. I went off the pill. We had a vague idea when I might be ovulating and after sex I would swing my legs above my head and practise water ballet – all good fun stuff you see in the movies. By the time I turned 35 we realised getting to the second act – a positive pregnancy test – might be harder than we thought. Sperm tests, a laparoscopy and a few ultrasounds of all my bits later proved nothing was physically wrong with us. We were lumped on the great pile of confused couples with 'unexplained infertility'.

Our fertility specialist said it could be emotional, psychological or, more likely, something physical they just weren't picking up in their tests. In a way, this news was worse than having an actual diagnosis that could be fixed; it could be nothing, it might be everything. I spent the next year scouring Internet sites for more and more information on unexplained infertility. I worried, I nagged Ben into drinking zinc and giving up coffee, I turned up at work just to Google 'Why am I infertile?' or, on very bad days, 'Why am I freaking bonkers?' I forgot what I wanted from life (apart from a baby). I didn't want to socialise. I couldn't look new mums in the eye, let alone pregnant women – they were the enemy, conspiring against me, rubbing it in. I was being unreasonable and unfair – I know! It was as if I had entered a different world and while I knew in my heart there were others out there just like me, it was a lonely place.

A few months before I turned 36 our fertility specialist convinced us to do a round of IUI (Intrauterine Insemination) where they squirt your partner's spruced-up 'washed' sperm directly into your uterus, giving it a head start on finding an egg. I crossed my fingers (and my legs) and prayed that this treatment would finally be the answer. But it didn't work. It suddenly hit us that nothing might work. Not IUI, not IVF. I knew Ben would be there at the end of the road but I wondered what I might be like when we got there. Bitter? Numb? Completely nuts? We reluctantly started looking into IVF as the logical next step and penned in our first consultation for a few months' time. I'd never felt more out of whack with my body (the enemy) and I felt old, tired and angry.

A few weeks before my birthday a friend told me about a couple of holistic healers in our town – let's call them the Fertility Sisters – who had helped her to get pregnant a few years earlier. It only took one visit for them to uncover something I had buried all the way down behind my left fallopian tube – *maybe this is all in my head.*

'You can't *think* yourself pregnant,' they scolded me. 'You're so stressed! If you were a bunny rabbit the message you'd be sending your body is that there isn't enough green grass around to feed little bunnies. You have to leave your head behind – stop worrying, researching and even thinking – and move into your body and convince it that everything is fine, there's nothing to worry about, there's plenty of green grass, that it's the perfect time to have a baby. Oh, and take these very expensive supplements and juices that will turn your pee an interesting green colour.'

Bunny rabbits? Green grass? Aloe vera juice with phytoplankton?

It all sounded silly and, worse, even more out of control than what we'd already experienced with unexplained infertility. But for the first time in my life I felt completely useless. I couldn't fix this with my usual methods (stress and overanalysis). I needed a guru and the Fertility Sisters made a lot of sense (if I could just get the chanting right). I did everything they said to do that month and even Ben gulped down the liquid zinc, phytoplankton and pumpkin seeds. We promised to rela– sorry, chill out, and 'forget' about TTC (no one *actually* forgets, that's impossible!) and go back to our normal lives as best we could.

I did a lot of praying that month. I told my body over and over that this was the perfect time to have a baby. I imagined myself with a baby. I asked that little soul to come on down, already, because we were ready. We were ready! But instead of my usual military precision around ovulation time we happily abandoned my impossibly organised sex schedule. I started looking new mums in the eye again that month and tried to be happy for them. I also started writing this book as a way of helping others, just like me. I went back to my life the way it was before I became *obsessed* by the idea of a baby …

I was pregnant three weeks later.

Looking back, I know I'm one of the lucky ones. The very, very lucky ones. I have friends who wait years and years to get pregnant, have multiple miscarriages and failed IVF cycles. And they all fight on, and on, to become mums. This book is for them. And for every woman who has spent any time wanting a child, crying over a negative pregnancy test and gnashing her teeth through yet another baby shower. I wish someone had pulled me aside at the very beginning of our TTC experience and said 'Everything is going to be okay'. Because even if I hadn't gotten pregnant when I did, Ben and I would have gotten through it and battled on somehow, together. I just couldn't see how strong we were at the time. I bet you're stronger than you think you are. And you're in very good company.

Everything is going to be okay.

PS: No-one is allowed to relax during the reading of this book. Stop relaxing immediately. Do not relax! Nobody even say 'relax'!

ABOUT THE AUTHOR

Genevieve Morton was born in 1972 and grew up on a farm in Victoria, Australia. She now lives in Tasmania with her husband Ben, their son Rafferty and three charismatic chickens. When she's not at her computer she is in her wellies sighing at weeds in her vegetable patch. Before becoming a full-time mum and freelance writer Genevieve was a lifestyle reporter and columnist for many years at Australian newspapers the *Mercury* and *Sunday Tasmanian*. She has travelled and worked all over Australia and career highlights include picking tobacco with a mouthful of dirt and wrapping mangoes in fancy doilies in Queensland. Genevieve has had two feature film scripts funded for development through Screen Tasmania. The first was called *Saturn's Return* and the second, *June, July, August*. Both are romantic comedies. You can find *Bump & Grind* on Facebook and all are welcome to chat about trying to conceive and share information.

Genevieve is currently working on her next book, while aiming to finish a hot cup of tea and get out of the house without pumpkin mash in her hair.

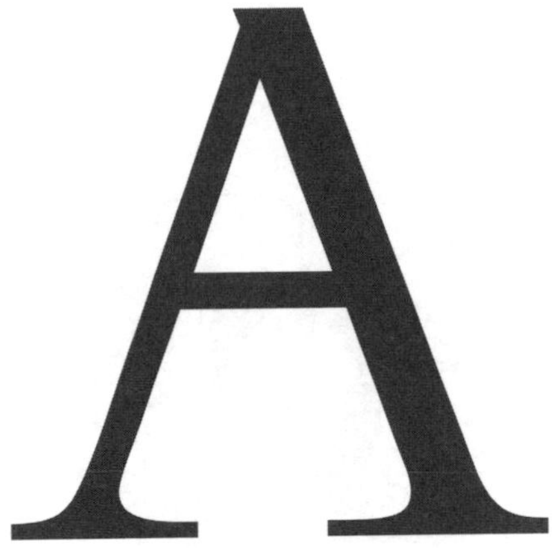

A is for another one!

It seems the minute you decide to have a baby one of your friends will pop out of nowhere excitedly panting 'I. Am. With. Child.' It can be annoying. Especially when you're dealing with a Smug Fertility Goddess who can be heard bragging that her husband 'just brushed past' her in the hallway and now she's pregnant while you've been body

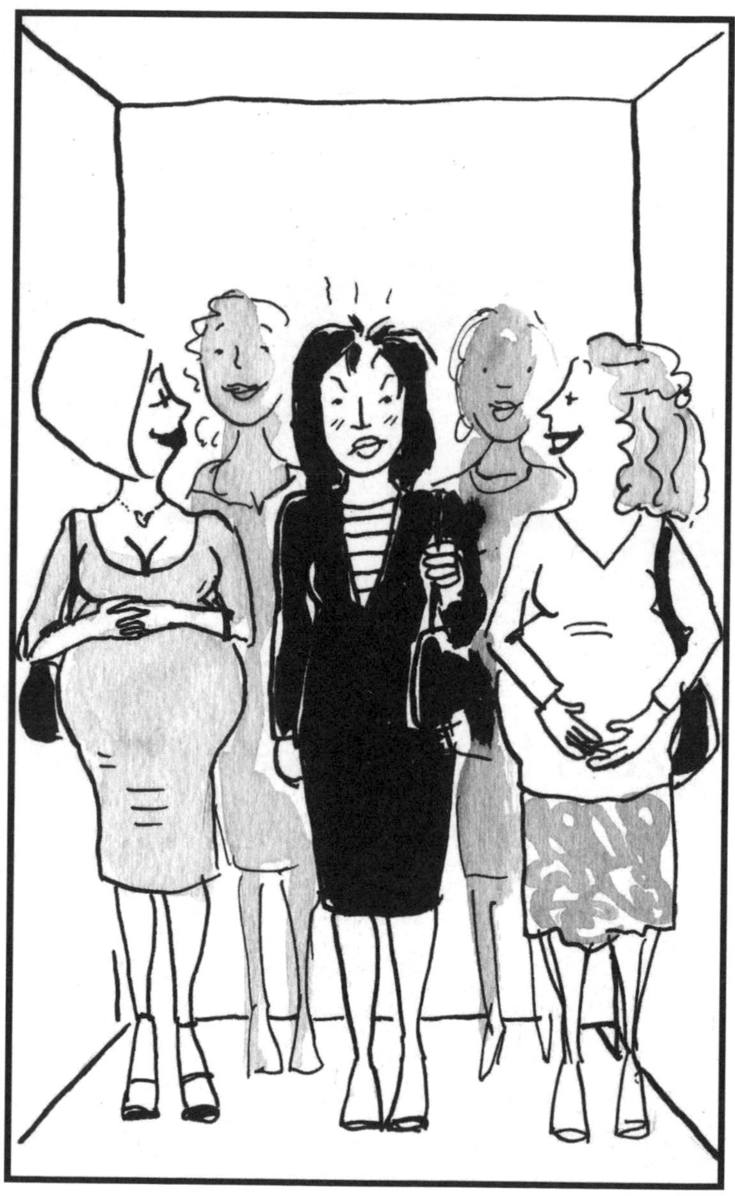

slamming your husband so keenly you could hold your own in a mosh pit.

Few things are more upsetting to the TTC community than news that *another* one of our friends, a celebrity and the lady who makes our coffee on the way to work are knocked up, up the duff, sprogged up, pregnant. It's almost impossible not to feel frustrated you're not popping the folic acid yourself and sharing your own happy news. The really big question we ask ourselves when we're TTC is 'Why not me?' You've probably given up booze, taken your temperature so many times you can do it in your sleep and had sex so many times you probably *are* doing it in your sleep. So, how come all the grind and no baby bump? Then there are the niggly, negative thoughts we have about ourselves when we ask 'Why not me?' Is it because I'm in my mid-thirties? Or is it because I'm no longer 'relaxed' about this? (Grrr!)

A little perspective.

The magical number 25

Almost all of us know the prime-time age for fertility in women is about 25 years. Women 25 or under have a 96 per cent chance of conceiving in a year, an 86 per cent chance between the ages of 25 and 34, and then it drops again in your late thirties. But who was ready for a baby at 25? Most of us hadn't met the right guy, established a career or learnt to stop drinking after three glasses of Chardonnay at that stage in life. For so many of us it was the *worst* time to have a baby. When we read the stats on women and age when it comes to baby-making there's an unwritten assumption that women somehow knew all of this and recklessly didn't sprog up in their mid-twenties anyway. Not true. I didn't give baby-making a second thought until I was 34 and (finally!) with the Right Guy. Lots of us meet the Right Guy in our late twenties or early thirties but need time together just as a couple before deciding to start a family. Many consider the thirties the happy medium age for motherhood: you're probably secure in yourself, your career and your relationship and you still have plenty of get up and go – without the Passion Pop. For me, the timing just felt right to start a family in my mid-thirties, and not a year sooner.

Some stats: The average British woman is now having her first child at 29 years of age. According to the author of the book *Fit For Fertility*, Dr Michael Dooley, one in every five American women is now having her first baby after the age of 35 – a 50 per cent increase on the last decade. 'Although a woman's fertility will start to decline from the age of 30,' he says, 'this does not mean you will automatically find it difficult to conceive.'

Overall, when you're in your thirties you have about a 15 per cent chance of getting pregnant in any given cycle. We all age individually too. And you can put the brakes on the ageing process with a rapid lifestyle overhaul (read on). Extra goods news is that women aged 35–39 are reportedly most likely to have twins even without fertility treatments, which raise the odds of multiple births. As you get older the level of your follicle stimulating hormone (FSH) increases, which ups your chances of releasing more than one egg each month. Hey, it happened to three friends of mine! They were all aged 36 and went on to have healthy, beautiful twins. Two for the price of one! But seriously, we can't worry too much about the Age Thing. Sure, there's no time to delay but you wouldn't have picked up this book if you were in the umming and ahhing stage anyway.

Here we are – whatever our age. Let's just go for it.

The relax factor

I'm not going to say the R word out loud but no, there is no evidence to suggest that moderate amounts of everyday stress will adversely affect your fertility. You can rela– sorry, chill out about that right now. However, there is something in having a happy heart and healthy body that will help things along and just make the TTC process a whole lot easier. But we'll get to all that good stuff a bit later …

For now, another one of your friends is packing up her ovulation predictor kit and moving to Mummyville. So what do you do? You take a deep breath, count to three, and ...

Storm out?

If the news Another One is expecting turns you into a blubbering mess or makes you gnash your teeth so hard your husband can hear you from the next room, you might want to get out of there. Perhaps excuse yourself amid all the squealing over the mum-to-be and spend some time in the bathroom getting yourself together (or messing up her fancy soaps). In a quick poll of TTC friends, the second most irritating aspect of trying, closely trailing behind being told to 'relax', is when a friend goes from TTC to triumphant. The normal reaction is that of anger, jealousy and wanting to run a very, very long way away from her.

> 'When my best friend told me she was pregnant I was so overcome with jealousy and shock I sat in silence for five minutes and then started sobbing. I had a big smile fastened to my face the whole time and kept saying 'Wow, great!' over and over. I pretended I had a stomach ache and my husband took me home.' **Cath, 34**

If there's no getting away, what do you say?

There's enough gushing over her baby news to warrant calling a plumber but there's no getting away from her. What do you say? You say all the things you're supposed to say! Just in case the green-eyed monster gets your tongue, here they are:

'I'm so happy for you!'

'You and What's-His-Name must be so excited!'

'When is the baby due?'

'Wonderful, wonderful news.'

And here's what you're secretly allowed to think:

'Hope it doesn't get What's-His-Name's nose.'

'You might want to lay off the chardonnay, love.'

'Duh, the sperm found the egg, it happens!'

'Crap, crap news, why isn't it happening to me?'

Why your partner won't understand the tears

Not long after you make your escape, the angry tears or bolts of indignation can seem to come out of the blue. They used to come to me during the car ride home. 'But she wasn't even planning to have a baby!' I'd cry. 'Isn't she too into her partying to get pregnant anyway? It's not fair! I've been living on pumpkin seeds for a year!' My husband Ben didn't understand the tears at first. He thought that because we were trying to get pregnant the news of other women's pregnancies would be reassuring – if she can then we can. He was wrong. Their news just made me jealous and sad and then annoyed with myself for being angry and self-obsessed – why couldn't I just be happy for her?

I had to start prepping Ben for incoming TTC breakdowns about a year in. 'If someone announces they are pregnant at this party then I'll probably cry all the way home,' I'd say. He eventually understood that being angry was just a downside of TTC when Another One got lucky. Yes, I was happy for the latest friend to make the announcement but I was also inconsolably upset that we weren't there yet. In the end I let Ben off the hook and told him he'd never really understand what it felt like for me in those car rides home – because he couldn't – and that was okay. He just had to be there for me and give really, *really* big cuddles when we got home (he got good at those!).

> 'The minute we decided to have a baby everyone around me seemed to fall pregnant and it felt like every second woman in the street had a tiny baby in her arms. Even my neighbour's cat got pregnant in the 10 months we were trying. The cat's good news pissed me off too!'
>
> **Lesley, 30**

Dodging another one

When you've been TTC for a while, being around newly pregnant women can swing between mildly irritating and wildly annoying. It's a pretty selfless and sturdy woman who doesn't have at least a pang or two of 'Oh puh-lease!' when Another One gets lucky before she does. Sometimes it can feel so much better when we put down the politeness and step away from the obligatory niceness.

Here's how you *could* handle it.

Lie

Have you noticed how work these days is the ultimate Get Out of Everything Free card? Bogus but cleverly crafted work excuses will get you out of most weekday social catch-ups, weekend lunches, even afternoons with the relatives if it's a recently pregnant sister or sister-in-law you can't face. Being busy is the new black so try it on to get you out of social engagements where Another One or a Smug Fertility Goddess might be lurking just ready to slap you with an ultrasound. TTC is undoubtedly a sneaky, private and very calculating time (and that's just the sex!). If you want to be crafty too, here are some bogus concoctions I prepared earlier: you have drinks with work friends, you've promised to see a movie with your partner, you have to work late, you have a work project to finish on Sunday or, when none of that comes to mind, you're not feeling well. Don't be afraid to protect the most important person in the room with a few white lies – that's you!

'32 was the age most of my girlfriends all seemed to get pregnant. It was the loneliest year of my life because I just couldn't handle being around them without feeling sad and frustrated. When they called, I just said I was busy. I was so much happier not having to see them all the time.' **Kim, 37**

Be honest

Tell her how you feel. Explain that being around her – and other newly pregnant women – is a bit too painful right now and you'd rather not turn up to every Oh-My-God-I'm-Pregnant event. A good friend will understand and give you some space while probably being quietly disappointed she can't share more baby joy with you for a while. A not-so-great friend will be oblivious to your feelings, feel put out that you're not jumping for joy with her or even feel that you're ruining her joy and hold it against you.

It's up to you.

Personally, I was always sliding out of social engagements faster than you could say 'Pass me the lube'. If you don't want to catch up (again!) to debate if this baby-to-be is an Oliver or an Olivia with Another One then don't do it.

> 'Now that we're TTC I hang out more with my single friends who have no interest in babies. There's no pressure to talk about it! All my real fellow-desperate TTC friends are online.' **Sam, 33**

PS: You're allowed to be angry when you hear the news Another One got lucky. Kick things around (maybe not your husband). Get the anger out of your body and cry – it's better than bottling it up. It'll be you making that announcement soon! Plan now how you're going to bang on about it and bore everyone senseless.

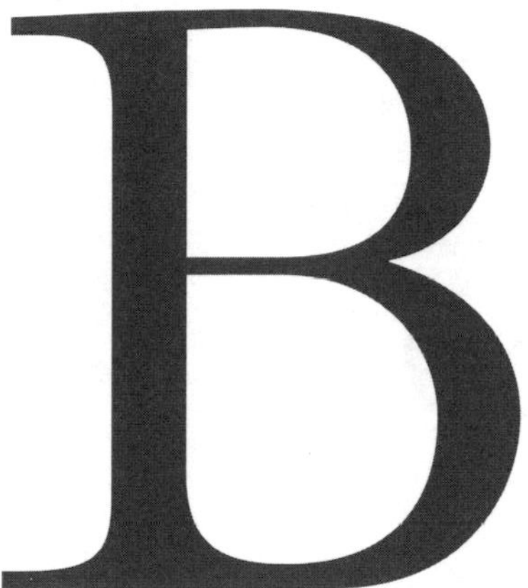

B is for Baby Gods

Ah, the Baby Gods with their infinitely mysterious and infuriatingly random decision making on who gets to sprog up and who doesn't. Let me tell you the story of Sue. Sue went through nine rounds of IVF in her mid-thirties without success. The strain on her marriage eventually found her divorced, and then, reluctantly, out there on the dating

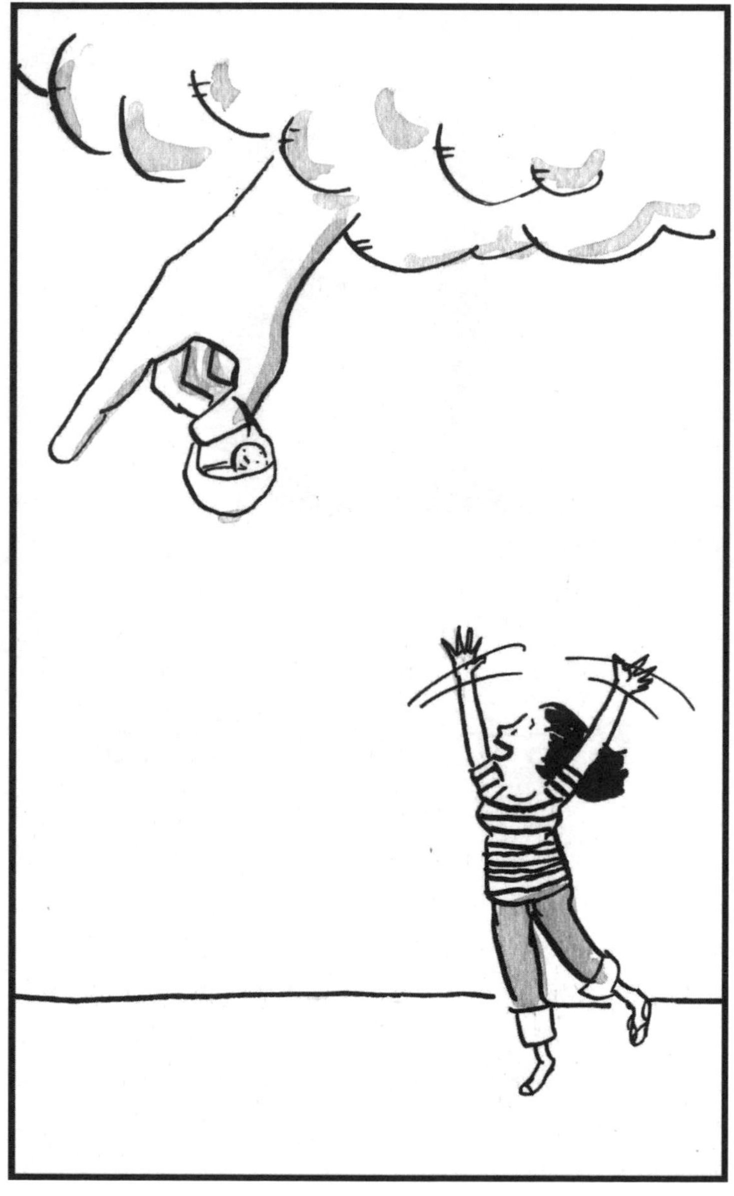

scene. One night when Sue was 40 she went out on a friend's mad hen night, got drunk and had sex with a bisexual man – using a condom – and *she got pregnant*. This is a true story. I kid you not. Sue went on to have a nice little boy called Daniel.

How does this happen?

While I'm happy for Sue, with all due respect it's because *the Baby Gods suck!* They really do. What seems like an impossible situation randomly ends in a pregnancy and what seems so likely – such as so many of us charting away our thirties with our legs in the air – does not end in a pregnancy (at least, not straightaway). During so much of my research for this book and time spent with my head in the oven, I heard 'It's not fair!' over and over. TTC is *not* fair and the Baby Gods are to blame. They are the mysterious and infuriating puppeteers in this great and unpredictable play called Knocking Oneself Up. Yes, your diet, timing sex, keeping the sperm spruced up, staying Zen and going through infertility treatment will all help your chances, but at the end of the cycle it is *still* in the hands of the Baby Gods.

That's why we're all going to make friends with the Baby Gods right now. I'm told it's healthier to have them onside from the very outset rather than screaming obscenities at them like I did every month when they failed to deliver.

How to kiss-arse with the Baby Gods

- Acknowledge that TTC is a tad out of your control and that's okay.
- Stop blaming yourself immediately.
- Stop being so hard on yourself.
- Let go of any expectations of what you thought TTC would be and accept your experience so far for what it is (it's about to get better!).
- Accept that your original TTC plan might change and keep an open mind.
- Promise now that you won't forget to *thank* those nasty Baby Gods when they deliver next month – but we'll get to that.

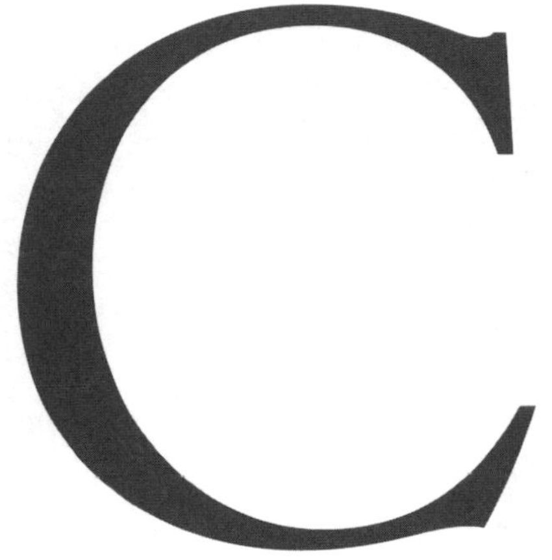

C is for confidante

Your partner is of course your closest TTC confidant but there does come a day (about the second) when listening to you bang on about cervical mucus will cause him to start losing interest, and probably his erection. That's when sisters and best friends come into play. They can offer the greatest support when you need them the most, especially if they've trodden this path before. But be very

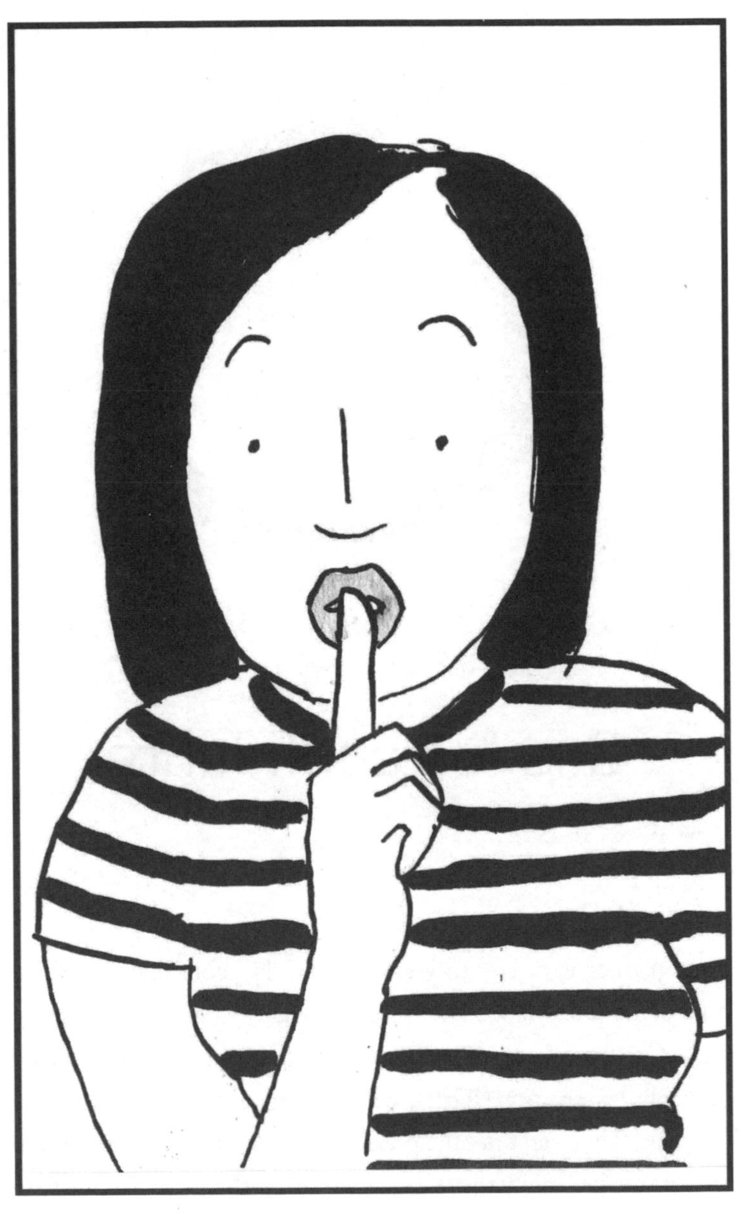

careful who you choose to share the absolute ins and outs of baby-making with. Some friends and relatives – despite their best intentions to be there for you – love talking about anything related to Other People's Problems and you don't want your fertility issues becoming fodder at their next dinner party.

I was lucky my sister and I were both battling the Baby Gods at the same time and we could spend hours on the phone discussing everything from acupuncture to our TTC-weary husbands. The most important thing was that I trusted her. I knew she'd be there for me to listen when I wanted to be sad and angry and I knew she'd be there for me when I didn't want to talk about it at all – not even with her. Trust and compassion are key.

The ideal TTC confidante is:

- someone trustworthy and kind
- someone who is *not* a Smug Fertility Goddess
- someone who can keep a secret (no matter how juicy)
- someone who will always be on hand to listen to you talk about your temperature dips and achey boobs (no matter how boring you get).

> 'Unknown to both of us my sister-in-law and I were both trying to have a baby at the same time and not having any luck. After a few too many drinks one night we started talking about it and both ended up in tears. We've been best friends ever since.' **Lesley, 30**

Telling people

Why not tell everyone you're TTC? Because they'll keep asking you how it's going and show nothing but enthusiasm, sympathy and then concern every time they see you and eventually you'll want to kill them for it. What if you've already told people you're TTC but now you want them to back off? That's easy. You come up with five infuriatingly vague responses to get you out of any discussion about it.

When anyone asks you 'Are you trying to have a baby?'

You reply with any of these:

'Oh, it's definitely on the To Do list, along with other stuff like – (insert boring house renovations or holiday plans)' until their eyes glaze over.

'We'll just see what happens. How are *you*?' (divert their attention)

'It'll happen when the time is right.' (very Zen)

'Oh yeah, baby-making stuff. We're not really thinking about it.' (blasé)

'I'm sure we'll let you know if – and when – we have anything to talk about.' (piss off)

Very effective, believe me! I have used all of them over and over. Good friends and sensitive types realise you're being vague on purpose and won't push you on it. Insensitive or clueless types might ask a few more questions or jump straight into offering unsolicited advice such as 'Well, you just have to stay relaxed!' or 'No use getting uptight about it, that won't help things along!' or 'You career girls, leaving it all so late!' To which you are allowed to make rude hand gestures and walk away.

> 'I feel like I can talk to most people about just about anything but when it comes to TTC and how secretly painful it is for me, I barely say a word.'
>
> **Heather, 36**

Why it's nice to have a confidante or two

For a while there I was keeping our flailing fertility a fiercely guarded secret. I didn't want people to know we were struggling with it because I feared their pity or, worse, useless advice like 'Just relax!' It wasn't until I got home from having a laparoscopy – where they stick a tiny camera inside you to check out all your reproductive bits and pieces – that I realised I might *have* to talk to someone. A good friend called me to see why I'd been away from work for the week and while she knew we were trying to have a baby she didn't know how *hard* we were trying and what I was going through to get there. On hearing I was recovering from day surgery she said she was sad we seemed to be having trouble getting pregnant. I kept saying 'It's okay, it's okay!' but I was crying through the words. *It wasn't okay.* I soon started confiding in her about how much TTC was getting to me, how frustrated and scared I was. It felt good to say these things out loud (finally!) and I knew she wouldn't talk to anyone else about it.

> 'My husband said I was 'obsessed' with TTC so I stopped talking to him about it. He mostly thinks we've 'stopped trying'. He doesn't even catch on that I molest him once a week every month and then not at all for weeks.'
>
> **Kate, 28**

It doesn't matter who your confidante is just so long as you trust them and they're compassionate and kind. If your best friends or sisters don't quite cut it, talk to your favourite neighbour or a family friend. You'll know who your true confidante is by their response to your first initial TTC talk. If they start relating your woes to their own situation and bypass your feelings and concerns then it might be wise to avoid them. If they listen to your story offering nothing along the lines of 'It was so easy for us!' or 'It'll happen when it's meant to!' then you may have a true confidante. If they listen, offer support and reassurance, if they cheer you up and constantly encourage you to keep going and stay positive – that's the confidante for you.

The whole 'friend in need is a friend indeed' concept is especially true in TTC. Anyone who has battled the Baby Gods and won the fight wants other women to stick it to the Baby Gods too. Your confidante will want to help you in any way she can – even if that's just listening. And listening. And listening …

Quick Quiz: Could you be driving your confidante crazy?

1. Do you start all your conversations with 'So I took my temperature this morning and…'?
2. Do you stare into space when talk strays from your cycle?
3. Do you ask your confidante things only a doctor might know?
4. Have you ever asked her to assess the size of your boobs in the Two Week Wait or – oh no – the colour of your nipples?

If you answered 'yes' to most of the above then yes, your confidante knows enough about you to put your old diaphragm to shame. If you answered 'no' to most of the above then the only person you might be driving crazy is you! Hurrah!

PS: You will find lots of confidantes to talk to online but we'll get to them in 'I is for Internet angels'.

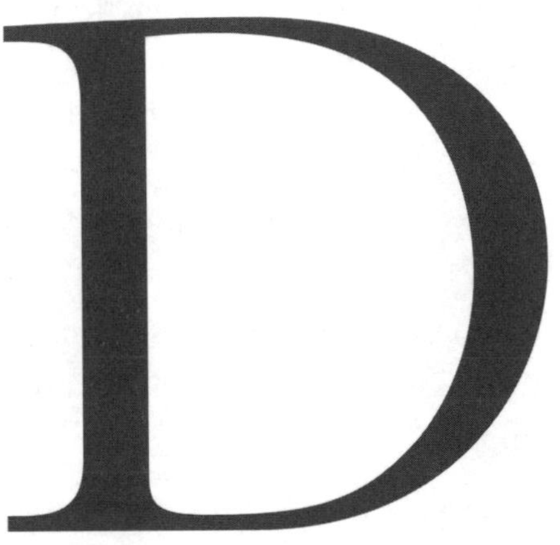

D is for daddy

Oooh, that's right! There's a daddy in this baby-making business! He's the one you're about to share your genes with so let's hope they're a good fit. So what's this daddy-to-be like? Does he remind you to take your folic acid? Does he say 'Don't worry honey, it's day 21, don't you get out of bed,' or 'I love it when you get so determined to have a baby you

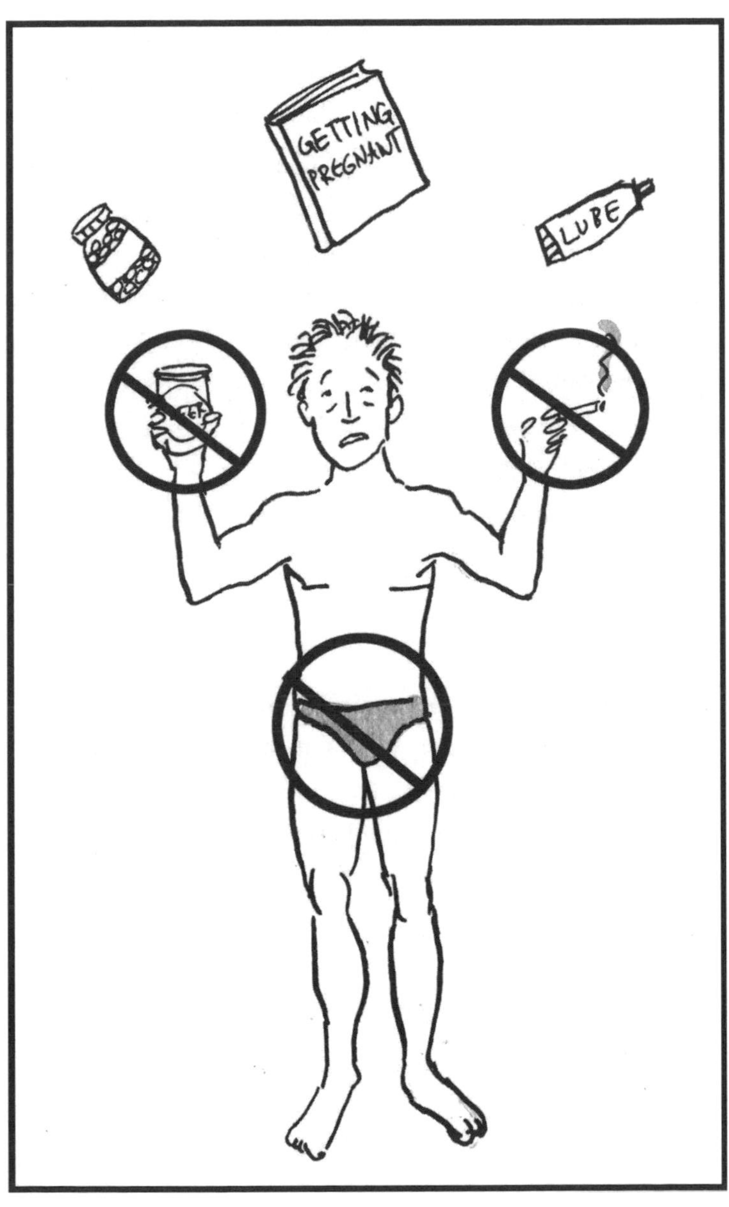
GETTING PREGNANT
LUBE

spend the day crying in the bathroom and shouting at me, it's so cute!'

Hmm, didn't think so.

I learnt pretty quickly that while Ben wanted to be there for me and do whatever he could to help me get pregnant (aside from the obvious!) he didn't want daily updates on my cycle. He stopped *actively* listening somewhere between 'Maybe I need more vitamin B6' and 'Oh God, I'm heading into menopause!' And fair enough. Guys just don't approach TTC the way we do. We like to research, examine all the facts and compare with our online TTC friends or confidantes. Most men just want to know the basic facts, when to have sex and some quick fixes should anything be wrong. That's why I've written a Daddy TTC Cheat Sheet for you to show him directly. But first …

Quick Quiz: Are you a TTC nag?

1. When your partner walks out the door to play sport do you call out 'Take care of your tackle'?
2. When he orders a second coffee do you roll your eyes and ask 'Are you sure?'
3. Have you thrown out all his tight undies and Speedos?
4. When he goes out with mates do you instruct him to only have three beers – no more?
5. Do you reschedule his social life around ovulation?
6. Do you force him to leave work early to 'service' you?
7. Do you bribe him into having sex even though he's clearly not *up* for it?

If you answered 'yes' to most of the above then your nagging/coaxing/bribing is now considered foreplay (lucky guy!). If you answered 'no' to most of the above then you should congratulate yourself on the restraint you've shown thus far regarding the sperm dispenser, sorry, your partner.

How to stop nagging and still get what you want

- Throw out all his tight undies and fill his drawer with new easy breezy ones.
- Don't assume he's making TTC mistakes until it's obvious (stay out of the spa!).
- Put his supplements somewhere obvious so he doesn't have to think too much about taking them.
- Convince him he's never looked better since cutting down on booze.
- Don't verbally nag for sex, just go for his pants.
- Don't alert him to which day it is in your cycle every five minutes (so not a turn on).
- Make sex dates and times you both agree on.
- Make sex dates fun – not too business-like.
- Allow him to have a life outside TTC.
- Allow him lifestyle slip-ups and try not to get too grumpy.

What he's going through

Guys generally want to fix problems but most of the time with TTC unless it's a sperm problem, he won't be able to.

He might feel frustrated it's not working as quickly as it does in the movies or for his friend Dave (who smokes way more weed than your guy does). He's probably also worried about how worried *you* look sometimes. He'll try to understand when you nag and cry and look depressed every time you get your period but unless he has a womb, he just won't ever truly get it. He might get annoyed after a year when you're still whining about the amount of coffee he drinks or if he should have gotten so smashed at the office Christmas party.

If he's been told his sperm is 'normal' then most guys assume their lifestyle is just fine and you can feel like you're banging your head against a wall when he comes home from the gym after using the steam room or worse, the sauna (puh-lease!). We women often feel as if it's full-on TTC or nothing but a lot of guys still want to live their lives as normally as possible and 'see what happens' without all the stress and pressure. And that's fair enough. But there is a nice balance between productively TTC *and* living his life. It's about understanding what The Fellas down there need – and most importantly what they don't need.

'I could nag for Britain if it were an Olympic event when it comes to my partner and TTC. All his mates with kids drink a lot and smoke so he just won't believe it's that bad for sperm. It's an ongoing battle.' **Deb, 34**

The sperm game

A-grade sperm needs to fulfill three components: quantity, quality and motility. No matter how sure a man is that his sperm is just as burly and fired up as he is to get the game won, sometimes it's just a big girl's tea party down there – which is fine. They just need better coaching.

Quantity: You want 20 million of those bad boys in their footy boots with their socks pulled up per millimetre of semen. Of the millions ejaculated, only about 200 will reach the egg in your fallopian tube. And only *one* special player is needed to fertilise the egg and kick the winning goal (no pressure!).

Quality: Along with having good numbers, you want them to have good shape and structure (morphology). The World Health Organization says 15 per cent or more of normal sperm constitutes normal fertility. That is, an oval head and a long tail that propels it forward. Sperm with large, small, tapered or crooked heads or kinky, curled or double tails are generally on the sidelines cutting up the oranges.

Motility: Good looks and plenty of friends will only get sperm so far. To reach the egg, each sperm has to move on its own, swimming and wriggling its way forward. You want at least half of the sperm on the field moving.

Of course, you can't tell any of this by looking at the line-up, no matter how hard and fast they tumble onto the pitch to play (just let me know when the footy analogy wears thin!). To really get to know the team you have to have a basic semen analysis test at a fertility clinic – but we'll get to that in 'G is for getting on with tests and treatment'. Don't be afraid. Don't be afraid at all.

For now, what are the obvious nasties that reduce quantity, quality and motility?

The sperm wars

Smoking: Men who smoke may have misshapen sperm which may move slower than the sperm in non-smokers. Smoking also damages DNA. Research shows men who smoke and drink alcohol have lower sperm counts and motility than men who are health nuts (nuts being the operative word here).

Booze: Heavy drinking reduces the quality and quantity of sperm. Alcohol may result in abnormal liver function and a rise in oestrogen levels that can interfere with sperm development. Up to two standard drinks a day is considered fine. If he's already had the sperm tested and his count was low, he should try abstaining from all booze for up to three months (because it takes sperm three months to develop) and test again.

Weed: Smoking marijuana decreases FSH (follicle stimulating hormone), LH (luteinizing hormone) and testosterone while increasing prolactin in the body, resulting in impaired sperm creation, function and motility. Sperm in a weed smoker reportedly goes too hard too fast and then dies out quickly before getting anywhere near the egg. Cocaine and opiates can also contribute to erectile dysfunction and amphetamines decrease sex drive. Your partner might want to stay away from those too.

Hot tubs: Spending more than 30 minutes in water 40°C or above may lower sperm count. Same goes for saunas and steam rooms.

Keeping cool: Fertility specialists call it 'increased scrotal temperature' and tight undies, sitting for long periods at a time (such as at a desk or behind the wheel), the use of laptop computers (in your lap) and too much bike riding will all give your partner a smokin' hot groin area – but not in a nice way. Ideally the temperature of your partner's scrotum should be 4°C lower than the rest of his body.

Tight little undies: Somewhere between Y-fronts and boxer shorts men discovered snug little pants that are to sperm what kryptonite was to Superman (hmm, he wore snug briefs over his tights too!). Alas, many men are reluctant to make the journey back to good old flappin'-in-the-wind boxer shorts and nice baggy, breezy Y-fronts. As a gift to Annoyed Women Trying to Sprog Up Everywhere many companies now sell cute semi-snug undies that won't strangle The Fellas during the day. They're like a tight version of boxer shorts with a wide elastic band up top and a nice flappy Y-front out in front. They're in all department stores – just don't buy them in too small a size! At night, tear off those undies and force him into good old-fashioned boxer shorts or even better, nothing at all. Instead of nagging your man into finding the right undies for the job, buy them for him and line them up in his closet. Men don't like being told what to wear and what to do (blah, blah) but when it comes to this one he just has to trust you and try to hang loose.

> ‘I even stopped my husband using our electric blanket when we were TTC because I heard the heat could damage sperm. The poor guy would sleep naked in the cold. Devotion!’ **Karen, 38**

Forcing supplements into him

A TTC friend of mine loves telling me the story of her husband who griped about taking his three supplements a night. It was an effort to remember, he said, he couldn't be bothered, what a hassle. Meanwhile, she was injecting herself every night for IVF! Instead of letting her husband off the hook with the supplements, she treated him like a three-year-old and dished them up with a glass of milk with his dinner every night. She used that horrible mocking tone we women adopt when we're being funny/serious (they hate that!). He soon learnt to take his own supplements – without the grizzling – and the milk and the mocking stopped.

For the rest of us, put his supplements somewhere obvious. Guys aren't obsessed with TTC and they do genuinely forget these things. Put them next to his cereal box or next to his bong – sorry his juicer. He'll need a good quality multivitamin and a zinc supplement (you can buy this from a health food shop) that you can keep in the fridge. Alternatively, you could look into a one-stop supplement for him designed especially for men to enhance their fertility. Ask your pharmacist to recommend a good one. The best thing to do would be to both go and see a naturopath, preferably one who specialises in fertility management, for a complete guide to supplements, with your special needs in mind. That way you can have your diet and lifestyle assessed too. Your guy might be making a simple mistake – such as having too much caffeine or alcohol – which can be quickly corrected.

The good news

With a good game plan – diet, exercise, not too many toxins, the right supplements and boxer shorts – your partner can dramatically increase the quality, quantity and motility of his sperm in no time. When you're TTC, sperm should be 'refreshed' (that is, ejaculated out) every three days or so throughout the entire month. In other words, don't save up a week's worth for ovulation. You want fresh, keen players ready to go. Saved up sperm can be sluggish and, well, half dead – and who wants them on your team? Flush those losers out and make way for new recruits. There are exceptions to the rule, of course, on saving up sperm if your partner has been tested and he has a low sperm count. Only your fertility specialist can tell you if you have a low sperm count. (See 'G is for getting on with tests and treatment.')

What happens if he changes his mind and wants a break from TTC?

In a very biological sense, he does hold all the power – you need the, er, gizz. But you don't want to have a baby without him emotionally onboard, right? You wouldn't trap him into a pregnancy (although I've heard of women pin-pricking condom packets in the hope some sperm will get through). You want him 100 per cent into the idea. So what happens when he changes his mind? Do you nag him into changing his mind back? Offer up emotional blackmail? Back off until he (hopefully) changes his mind back on his own?

'Respect and communication are important here. It is important to know if your husband's suggestion is based on his need for a break or because he thinks you need a break, despite what you think. If your husband says he needs a break it is important to respect that, especially as he probably wanted a break last time but held in there for one more cycle, for your sake. If he thinks you need a break allow him to give you feedback, listen 'til he finishes and then thank him for caring so much. Take some time away from the topic before you discuss it further.'

Psychologist and IVF counsellor, Lynne Quayle.

Blokey reasons for a change of heart

- He's not ready (emotionally).
- You're both not ready (financially).
- He's scared (it's a big decision).
- Work is full-on (and he wants to keep home life easy).
- You're getting 'obsessive' about TTC and he just wants to 'be' for a while.

> 'If anything, my husband is more baby-mad than I am! He's the one who gets uptight about my cycle and what we should be doing to conceive. He's a freak, I know.' **Sam, 33**

It's not easy to take a break from TTC when your ovaries are clanging so loud you could form your own rock band, but perhaps the best way to approach it is to resist getting angry. He's probably not changing his mind to hurt you. Talk about *why* he has changed his mind. Don't confront him the minute he walks in the door with 'We have to talk about this!' (they find that one scary). It might be best to approach the subject when you are both calm, happy and not in super-serious mode. Perhaps tell him you're not going to get angry and upset, you just want to hear where he's coming from. Then actually listen. Really listen. Ask questions. Listen some more. Do you understand where he's coming from? Is it fair enough? Sometimes just listening and going back to a place of friendship with each other is enough. He may need to vent his fears and concerns before being reassured. He may just need some room from you to take TTC a little slower – or just be less intense about it. Then he'll come around.

Or not.

A friend of mine watched her husband do a complete back-flip on wanting a baby after a few months of trying. The idea of starting a family suddenly terrified him and she was understandably heartbroken. What did she do? She stayed for a while and nagged and nagged hoping he'd buckle under pressure. And then when that didn't work she left him. He wasn't going to come around and she, at 35, felt that she had to move on (don't worry, she met a great guy and went on to have a beautiful baby).

Most men *do* come around to it again, usually when their mate's wives are pregnant or they get a promotion at work and feel a bit more financially secure. Let him know what it means to you, how much you want to share the experience with him, that no one is *ever* really ready for a baby and that you'll promise to be patient – and not too nutso – with him while trying. Couples counselling might work if you want to be really proactive and he agrees to it. It might be a much deeper issue – such as his own feelings on childhood or family, or personal failings and fear he's not going to be a good father. These are important issues to discuss and for you to understand. It would be better to have them out in the open now, before any children appear on the scene.

Talking it all out – without anger and with lots of understanding – will help, and bring you much closer together.

> 'When my partner decided we needed a break from trying to make a baby I freaked out. It was the end of the world. Looking back he was just scared that it was *all* we were becoming – the TTC couple. I let it be for six months and then I said 'It's now or never'. I wasn't proud of myself. But it worked.' **Ann, 29**

Who can he talk to?

What if he wants to talk to his mates or family about TTC but you want to keep it just between the two of you? Most TTC friends I've talked to tell me their guy lets *them* call the shots on who they tell and don't tell. They agree to keep it quiet (less pressure) and only tell the world they've been trying when they are a nice safe 12 weeks pregnant and popping the champers. But what happens when the champers doesn't get popped for six months or more?

Ben agreed to keep our flailing fertility a secret at first but a year or so into TTC his mates started wondering why every now and then he'd abstain from all alcohol and coffee. I – kind of selfishly – thought he didn't need to vent his frustrations with them; after all, he had me to talk to. But keeping quiet wasn't really his style. He was used to confiding in people close to him about big stuff.

However, just as when you're choosing your own confidante, ask him to choose wisely. Not just for your own privacy but for his own sake too – you don't want his friends teasing him about 'firing blanks' and offering to 'do the job' for him.

What can he say when everyone asks *him* if you're trying to have a baby?

Guys feel the pressure too! No doubt he gets asked if the two of you are trying or when he's going to fulfill his duty (yuck) and impregnate The Missus (double yuck). Usually the best approach is for him to keep it light and evasive. Make jokes, divert the attention, change the subject (guys are good at that!).

> 'My guy had the best response when people harassed him about me not being pregnant. He'd just say 'When I find a good reason to put another person on the planet, I'll let you know.' That shut them up!' **Lynne, 39**

Daddy cheat sheet (hand over to your man)

Yes, your partner has just handed you a book that looks kinda girlie, possibly in the self-help area. Don't be alarmed. She's been acting a little kooky lately, for sure, but she hasn't lost her mind (well, not quite). She just wants you to understand a few things about this whole baby-making business so you can knock her up fast. We know you don't want *all* the details.

So, here are some facts and a few quick fix-its for you to try.

Fact: A daily multivitamin helps provide selenium, zinc and folic acid, trace nutrients vital in sperm production and function.

Fix it: Get yourself a good multi and zinc supplement.

Fact: Stress interferes with certain hormones needed to produce sperm. Plus it can kill your sexual mojo at the end of a working week.

Fix it: Find your own way to unwind and do it regularly (no bingeing on booze!). Get regular exercise and try to leave work on time.

Fact: Caffeine can impair your body's ability to absorb iron and calcium, upset your stomach and make you anxious (and you thought that was caused by being forced to have sex with your wife when you have your parents staying!).

Fix it: Limit caffeine to 300mg per day. That's three cups max of espresso coffee (lattes and cappuccinos). Caffeine can also be found in chocolate, cola drinks, energy drinks and tea.

Fact: Men who exercise to exhaustion show a temporary change in hormone levels and a drop in sperm quality.

Fix it: Don't go too hard at the gym. And forget about training for that triathlon when you're TTC. Save it for the bedroom.

Fact: Alcohol can cause the tubes that carry sperm to atrophy, loss of sperm cells and an increase in abnormal sperm cells.

Fix it: Cut right back to two to five units a week while you're TTC and don't save them all up to binge on the weekend! A 440 ml can of beer is 1.8 standard drinks. A standard glass of wine (25 ml) is 1.6 units, and a large glass (250 ml) is 3.3 units. You might just lose a few pounds and feel fantastic along the way.

Good luck!

But *they* got pregnant

Your partner might be wondering how his mate Dave knocked his wife up so easily when you all know he smokes a lot and drinks heavily. It might be a lot of factors. He might have a naturally high sperm count. He and his wife might do it right on ovulation every month. His wife might be the most fertile bunny who ever lived. They might have had a whole lot more sex than you. It might just be that they are the lucky ones. TTC isn't fair and we know the Baby Gods *suck*. But improving your diet and following a game plan will dramatically improve your chances in no time. Besides, who'd want Dave's kids anyway?

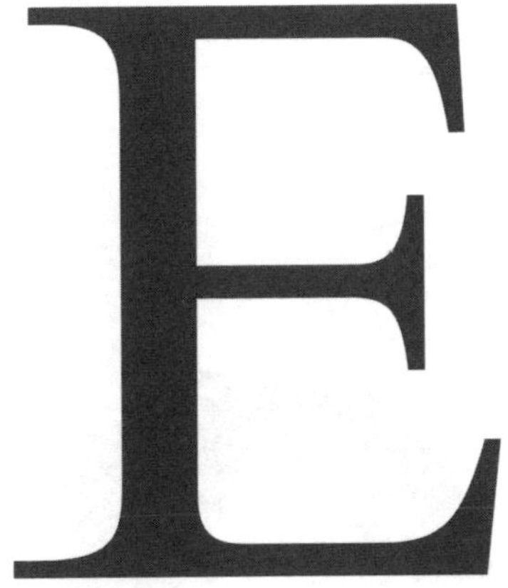

E is for everyone says ...

Everyone says 'just stop trying' and you'll get pregnant. Everyone says 'just get a puppy' and you'll get pregnant. Everyone says 'just take a romantic trip to Paris' and you'll get pregnant. Everyone says – well, who cares. You're probably sick of hearing what everyone says. Where does all this advice come from? Some of it from everyday urban

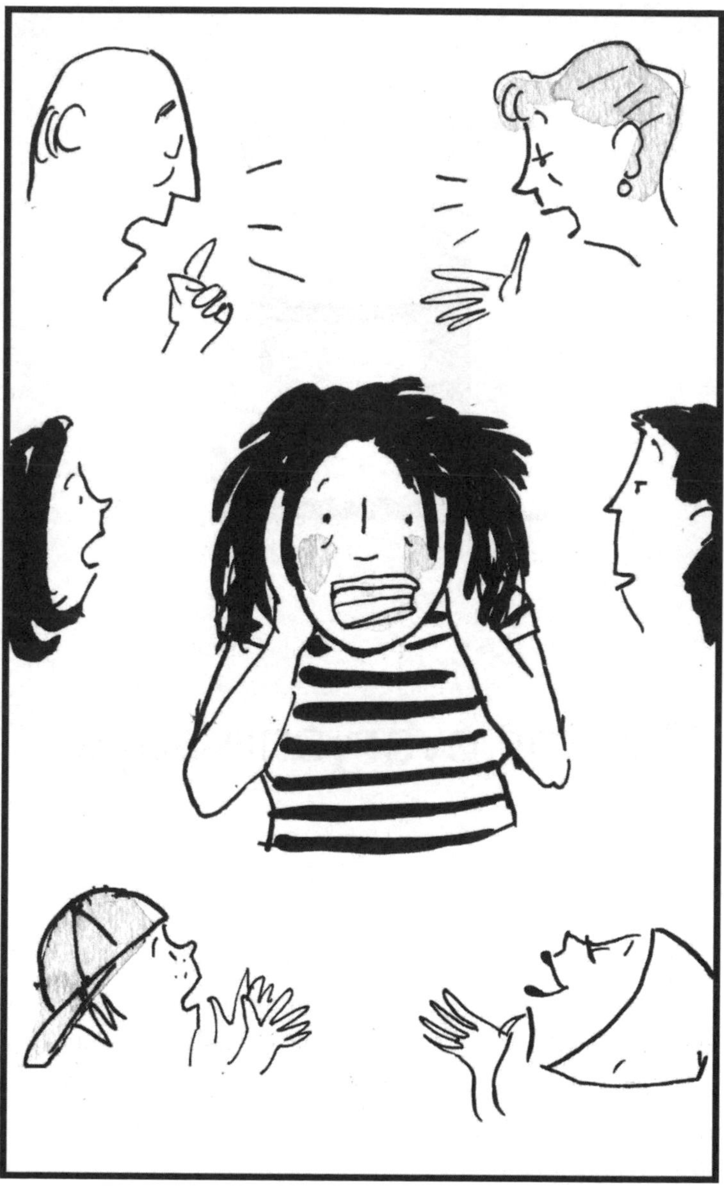

myth, some of it from ancient times and a little of it from your Aunty Barb who's been banging on about her fertility tricks for years. Let's go through the Top 10 Most Annoying Baby-making Myths and bust them, once and for all.

1. Just relax and you'll get pregnant!

The most irksome line ever uttered in the world of TTC. While it is true that lots of stress will cause your reproductive system to effectively shut down (it's part of that in-built fight or flight mechanism), there's no evidence to say that moderate amounts of everyday stress – such as that brought on when sprinting through the supermarket to avoid a Smug Fertility Goddess – will affect your chances of conceiving. The reason why it's so annoying (and there's a whole chapter on this: see 'R is for rela– don't say it!') is because it implies that only uber-Zen chilled out goddesses get pregnant and the rest of us moderately jumpy types miss out. It's just not true. Phew. Now you can rela– sorry, chill out about it.

2. Just get a puppy and you'll get pregnant!

I tried this one out and all I got was a whole lot of holes in the garden. Don't get me wrong I loved our puppy, but really, she was my pretend baby (with really big teeth). So many couples get a puppy when we're TTC because we want to experience 'parenting' and have a little life force depending on us. We were told a puppy was the wedge before a real live human baby and I desperately hoped so. Alas, puppies grow into dogs and eventually you realise you can't dress them in bonnets and booties forever (or the neighbours really will call the authorities and stop picking up your mail). Just be sure when you're buying a puppy that you're buying it for all the right reasons – and remember, you can't put a nappy on it.

'My husband bought me a puppy when we started IVF as a gift, just in case things didn't work out. They did work out – eventually! – and we have a beautiful little girl but we still dote on our dog, he was our first baby.' **Emma, 34**

3. Just adopt and you'll get pregnant!

According to Professor Robert Jansen in his book *Getting Pregnant: A compassionate resource to overcoming infertility*, there have been just five 'careful studies' on the chances of getting pregnant after adoption. 'In every one of these five studies,' states Jansen, 'it was obvious that couples who kept trying to get pregnant instead of adopting had more chance of conceiving than those who adopted!' He says that's because an adopted baby will actually *impair* chances of conceiving because the new baby's crying will interrupt your sex life. And yet so many people have success stories about couples they know who adopted and kapow! they got pregnant.

Why? Many experts say the *anecdotal* increase in women

getting pregnant after they adopt is because they simply give themselves more time to get pregnant. It might just take the same time to apply and adopt a child as to fall pregnant – a few years at least. It seems as if it 'just happened' when they adopted, but it might just be the time factor and even without the adoption they may have conceived naturally in that time frame anyway. Plus, for many, once they have adopted the pressure is off, they chill out, are happier and yep, that all helps conceiving too (I did *not* say 'relaxed'). So, it's no quick fix for fertility. Something to think about before we get all Angelina Jolie about things.

4. Just take a romantic trip to Paris and you'll get pregnant!

Because a ruddy croissant will clearly unblock your fallopian tube.

> 'My husband and I used to take TTC mini breaks around ovulation because everyone kept saying 'Just go on holiday and you'll get pregnant!' It didn't work for us. We conceived after really boring sex at home and I spent most of the weekend doing ovulation tests. I remember it being really stressful!' **Lesley, 30**

5. Just stop trying and you'll get pregnant!

But we have all the gear! The OPKs and the BBT charts.

Plus, my husband is so emotionally exhausted by all the 'trying' he's agreed to an Ovulation Week mini break!

Give up trying? I'm not sure anyone *genuinely* gives up. Perhaps couples inevitably stop being so hard on themselves (a good thing) and go back to their lives without TTC on their minds 24/7. But even then, TTC is usually lurking in the darkest corner of your mind, holding a little candle for you. There might be something in not trying quite so *hard*, but giving up trying altogether is almost impossible without using protection or going on strike (sexually speaking). When you are TTC you're trying, that's what the first T in TTC is all about. Just don't let it get too *trying*.

> 'It annoys me when people tell me they gave up and got pregnant. Did they really? Or did they simply pretend to give up and got lucky anyway because it was just their time?' **Karen, 38**

6. Just renovate your house and you'll get pregnant!

Maybe this one might work because your husband will suddenly look so sexy in his overalls you'll want to pounce on him between painting the kitchen and the living room. Or is it because you'll have to move out of your home because of the nasty paint fumes when you do get pregnant? Because life is full of wacky ironies like that, isn't it? Well, maybe. Get him to roll up his sleeves anyway. Maybe your fertility feng shui'd bedroom could do with a fresh coat of paint …

7. Just take a new job with a three-year contract and you'll get pregnant!

Why not take up kickboxing, pay for a trip around the world and get hooked on flaming sambuca shots? It's very tempting to want to challenge the Baby Gods with impossible situations, but you know in your heart that it won't matter what situation you're in when you get pregnant – you won't care, and work/life will just get shuffled around to accommodate your new circumstances. You don't want to disappoint a future employer by resigning or taking maternity leave soon after starting a new job, so perhaps for now just make life easier and stick with the job you have – better the devil you know – unless it really is time to move on.

8. Just spend a lot of time around other people's babies and you'll get pregnant!

This one used to work around the campfire in tribal times. If a woman was struggling to conceive she would spend lots of time holding other women's babies and her body would just naturally go into baby-making mode and start pumping out all the right hormones. When it comes to us – in present times – this of course depends on your friend's babies. There are the really wriggly, grabby ones that you just want to hand back immediately after they've stuffed a fistful of your hair in their mouth. Or those placid, dribbly ones that spew up their milk on your shirt which their mother then unwittingly wipes into your bra. Hmm. I'm not sure how long you'd want to hold one of those ...

9. Just stop thinking about it and you'll get pregnant!
You need a lobotomy before you can have a baby (well, duh!).

10. Just stop wanting a baby and you'll get pregnant!
Wanting a baby is *wanting* a baby no matter how old you are, whether you already have a child or you've just started swilling supplements and swinging your legs in the air. It's not something you can shut down or turn on and off. There is no playing hard to get with the Baby Gods (as much as we can try!). Pretending to stop wanting a baby is just telling yourself little fibs. Besides, you *deserve* to get what you want. You *deserve* a baby and you're going to get one too – and soon. There's nothing wrong with *wanting.* There might, however, be something in having other wants and desires too. You know, world peace and to fit into those skinny jeans circa 2007 …

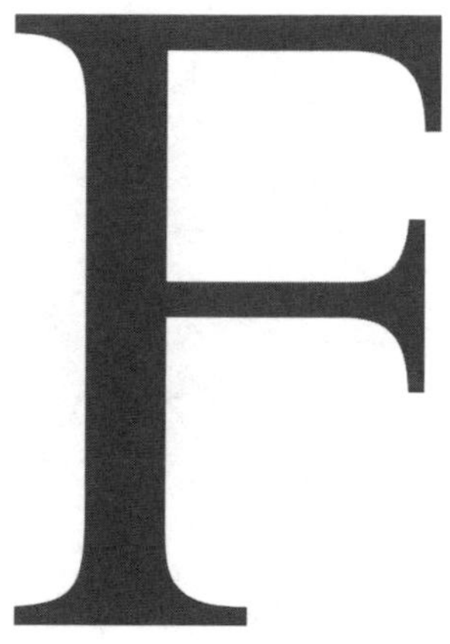

F is for friends and family

They mean well. They really do. But there's something about baby-making that brings out the Irritating Expert in most families and friendship groups. Maybe it's your mother-in-law who likes to trill that in *her* day getting pregnant 'just happened after you got married!' If I had a follicle for every time I've heard women aged over 60 say

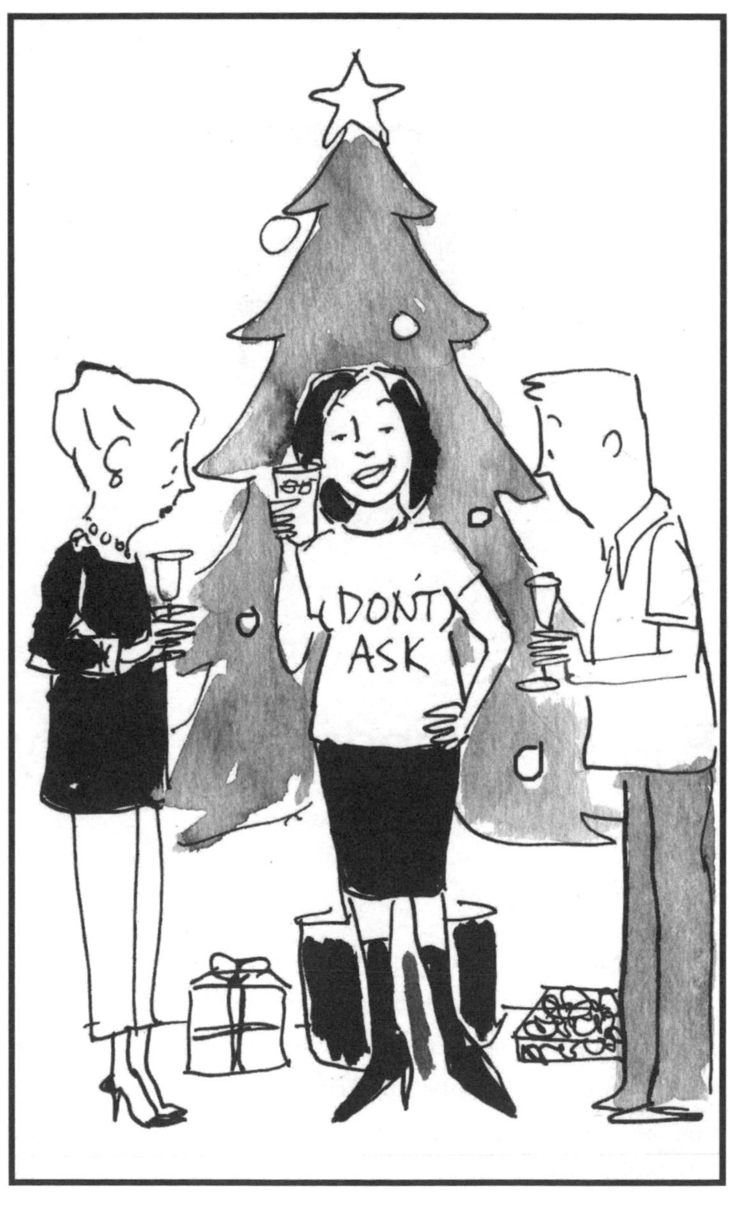
DON'T
ASK

'We just got married and had babies because that's what you did back then', as if what was expected of you somehow made it happen. If only!

Quick Quiz: Is your family driving you crazy?

1. Do any of your family members greet you with 'Anything yet?' as if you are waiting for the baby you bought on eBay to arrive?
2. Does your dad talk about 'Sterile Aunt Sally' who – tragically – couldn't have children, as his way of being 'understanding'?
3. Does your sister email you unwanted infertility information she Googles at work?
4. Does your mum quietly suggest your career is making you barren and perhaps if your husband left work on time or got a proper haircut he might be able to knock you up?

If you answered 'yes' to most of the above then it's time to relocate and start screening your calls. If you answered mostly 'no' then you have the sweetest, most considerate family ever. Can I take them home with me?

Mums

In *their* day they didn't seem to have too many problems getting pregnant, right? They didn't even think about it! The most obvious difference between their day and ours is that they were largely aged in their fertile-prime mid-twenties when they started baby-making.

It gave them a lot more time to get a little brood together. We know that the average British woman now has her first baby at 29. Those sweet days of starting your family in your mid-twenties are *over.* There's absolutely no point banging on about them.

'My mother-in-law literally called me every week to ask if I was 'having any luck' falling pregnant. I wished I'd never told her we were trying. I started screening her calls and eventually she got it and left me alone.' **Kim, 37**

Gran Central

All her friends are grannies. Your mum might be desperate to get her granny on too but until you sprog up, she can't. She might subtly ask you how baby-making is going, quietly suggest your career is the reason for – oh God no – leaving it all so late, or question the amount of hours your husband works and suggest that perhaps he's to blame. A granny-in-waiting needs to be carefully put in her place (and they can be sensitive!). If your mum is anything like the above then perhaps calmly tell her that you know she's keen for you to have a baby, but hearing how easy it was for her or her suggesting you 'relax' makes you uncomfortable/want to strangle her.

'My husband's mum sent me an expensive handmade baby rug as 'inspiration' to get pregnant after a year of no luck. As if that would help me! I let our cat sleep on it.' **Lynne, 39**

PS: It only takes one well-executed hissy fit to send your mum or mother-in-law packing. And don't worry, she loves you, she'll forgive you. She might even start to understand where you're coming from ...

Dads

Sweet, bumbling adorable dads – man, they can be annoying! They want to say the right thing ('I'm here for you') but they end up saying the wrong thing ('Your mother wants this so much for you').

Or, your dad won't know what to say and suddenly has your quest to have a baby right up there with religion and politics at the dinner table. Should anyone mention it he might swiftly change the subject and act as if he's doing you a favour. Which is fine. But if you want to talk about it, he's not. Plus, older men don't really want to hear about icky women's business such as ovulation, blocked fallopian tubes and cysts on your ovaries. And he definitely won't want to know about the highs and lows of your husband's latest semen analysis test – no matter how many beers he's had.

My dad did me the ultimate favour by simply not mentioning our baby quest for about six months, even though he did know we were secretly trying. Then one day out of the blue he gave me a big hug and told me I was going to be a great mum one day soon. I started crying and asked 'Really?' to which he looked surprised and said 'Of course!' That was all he needed to say.

> 'My dad is desperate to be a grandpa. He wasn't around for us kids much and I think he wants to make it up somehow. I feel that pressure.'
> **Kate, 28**

Those irritating hopes and dreams

Wouldn't it be nice if *some* parents paid more attention to what we have achieved already than to the wish list of things they want for us? It's sometimes not enough that we have a good relationship, a decent career and have stopped eating carbs after 3 p.m. It takes some gentle reminding to parents – no matter how old we are – that while becoming a mum yourself is right up there on your wish list too, it's not the *only* dream they can have for you.

Sisters

The best thing about sisters is that you can hang up on them then call back 10 minutes later and carry on as normal. They've seen you at your best, they've seen you at your worst, *and* they saw you the time you gave yourself a corkscrew perm back in the day. Sisters can make the greatest confidantes and the most wonderful friends when you're TTC. If you're close, you'll end up even closer.

My sister and I were lucky in that we were both embarking on the TTC journey at the same time. Somewhere at the very beginning we agreed not to push our own methods on the other and just support what the other one was going through. My sister started out very holistically by using acupuncture and a squeaky clean diet with all the right supplements. I started out very scientifically by charting my cycle and ignoring all my feelings. 18 months later my sister was embarking on IVF and I had turned myself into a super-spiritual bunny rabbit (read on). My sister says the most important thing about TTC is to accept that it may not go the way you'd planned. 'I thought IVF was the worst case scenario at the beginning,' she said, 'but 18 months later and after we had tried everything else, IVF was the most magical, wonderful thing that we were lucky enough to go into – after all, it worked.'

She agrees that when the TTC road twists and turns, sisters can offer the best support and even offer to take control of the wheel when things get too bumpy. I found out I was pregnant just eight weeks before my sister discovered she was pregnant too, after her first cycle of IVF. When I told her our pregnancy news on the phone I was really careful, not wanting to upset her because, as we all know, there is nothing worse than when someone goes from TTC to triumphant and forgets the road behind them. My sister was, without doubt, the happiest person in the world for Ben and I. I can still hear the squealing.

Dumb sister stuff

And then there's the dumb sister stuff that gets in the way of even the most holy of sisterhoods. Dumb sister stuff happens when we let our sibling rivalry turn us into green-eyed monsters and we torture our husbands during the car ride home from family events. Dumb sister stuff sometimes doesn't budge – no matter how old we get – but you can give yourself permission to *not* let it get to you this time. If you're the competitive type and your sister seems like your closest competitor, just remember: if you want to win, don't play the game. If she's too much to bear when she's pregnant then give yourself permission to stay away!

> 'My sister is younger than me and she has three kids that drive her crazy. She is envious of my life! It helps keep perspective on things as we keep trying. I can't help but gloat (loudly) about all my free time to myself!' **Anne, 29**

Brothers

Your brother's advice will no doubt stem from his partner's experience in TTC if they've already been through it. If she struggled to get pregnant then he might be sensitive about it and not question you too much or even offer encouragement and support. If his wife got pregnant after – oops – accidentally using his razor to shave her legs then please, cancel Christmas. You might not want to be around that guy.

The nice part is, brothers can be surprising. I eventually told my brother we were having problems getting pregnant and instead of offering blokey advice like 'Stand on your head' he just wished me luck and said he'd pray for me.

Not so sensitive brotherly types get it oh-so-wrong at all the wrong times. They sometimes use words like 'sterile' or 'barren' and – oh yes – 'frigid'. Who needs a family Christmas anyway?

> 'My brother said "Maybe you're infertile because you were a bit frigid at school." I wanted to *kill* him.' **Hannah, 31**

Educating family

The biggest problem many of us face when we're TTC is that you just can't hide from inquiring relatives. You can run but somehow no matter how far you go they'll still turn up at events to quietly corner you with 'So, I bet you'd love a family of your own' or 'You'll be next!' when your sister-in-law falls pregnant (again). You might just have to be honest about what you expect from them in this situation.

Most of them won't want to hurt your feelings and they have no idea they're being insensitive – people assume they're being 'helpful'. You might just have to calmly say that yes, you're trying for a baby but you don't want to talk about it and their advice and/or comments aren't wanted right now. If they want to help and support you and your partner then you will accept cash …

Of course, sometimes we need our family's help, especially if we already have a child and are going for another one through IVF or are just getting some tests done such as a laparoscopy, which does take about a week's recovery time. Parents are great at minding your little one when you need to see your doctor or can't get off the couch. A TTC friend of mine was very sneaky. She desperately needed the help of her nosey mother-in-law to look after her toddler while embarking on IVF. But when the mother-in-law got too close and insensitive about how IVF was progressing, my friend told her they were doing just one round – that was all. The first round didn't work and everyone – including the mother-in-law – backed off. But they did a few more rounds in secret and told all their parents afterwards – when they were a safe 13 weeks pregnant.

'Last Christmas, I got my period that morning so I had a few drinks during the day to cheer myself up. Unfortunately, they did the opposite and I *lost it* when my uncle suggested I better not leave having a baby too late. I went into a rant that turned into a big family fight. It just hit me all at once that people – men especially – just don't get it! They don't know how much it hurts when your family assumes having a baby is just a decision you make. It's so much harder than that.' **Anne, 29**

What to say to family (with a few white lies)

'We were trying but now we're giving it a break – all that sex!'

'I know you're curious but you'll just have to wait and see.'

'We're leaving it up to God to decide – we'll let you know when she does.'

'I know you're asking because you care but we're keeping that one private.'

'We're a bit too busy for babies this year.'

'Soon, soon, we have no plan, there's no rush.'

'We've decided to leave it for a while to renovate the house first.'

'Do they come with a warranty?'

'Isn't it enough that we all fuss over *your* children?'

‘If you are extroverts you can probably handle the full range of responses you will get. Quieter, more private people often find it very stressful handling questions and comments from others. I help these people become aware of their privacy boundaries and teach them how to be assertive with intrusiveness. You can say: “You might not be aware that I regard our fertility as private. I would appreciate it if we kept off the topic ... It feels like every time I see you, you ask about our TTC progress. While I appreciate your interest, can we leave it at that I will update you when I have good news?”’ **Psychologist and IVF counsellor, Lynne Quayle**

The problem with friends

If you're blessed enough to be surrounded by happy-go-lucky single friends who would rather lose their Jimmy Choos than have a baby then you're lucky. Hold onto those friends. But if you're like most of us then no doubt TTC talk comes up every now and then at social occasions.

The dumb things our friends say

'Just relax.'

'Go on holiday.'

'Don't think about it and it'll happen.'

'Have you been tested?'

'What position are you having sex in?'

'Are you doing it often enough?'

'You shouldn't wait too long – you're not getting any younger.'

'If it's meant to be, it'll happen.'

'Do you think you're subconsciously not ready for a baby so your body isn't giving you one?'

'Just do IVF – that always works!'

Ugh. Most of them have no idea what battling the Baby Gods is really about. That's why they openly complain about their children in front of you as you're secretly thinking they are incredibly lucky to have such lovely little ones. They just don't know. It seems to come down to an 'us and them' situation and it's as if you're living on different planets sometimes. The key is to explain things in very simple terms and be clear about what your personal boundaries are. You could say 'It's such a private thing I'd prefer not to talk about it' or 'I promise we'll let you know if we need your support but for now we're just keeping the whole baby thing really quiet'.

If you want to talk about TTC then let them know what a sensitive area it can be so please, tread carefully. If they want to support you, that's great. Here's a guide that might help them:

Don'ts for friends

- Don't ask how TTC is going in front of other people.
- Don't ask about TTC when I'm at work.
- Don't put me on the spot about TTC in front of other people – no matter how good a friend you think they are, talk to me privately.

- Don't ever suggest it might work if I a) relaxed, b) stopped trying so hard or c) had another glass of wine.
- Don't say you 'understand' if you haven't gone through a miscarriage or IVF – just listen.
- Don't tell me my possible pregnancy symptoms are 'all in my head' – just support me.
- Don't tell me to 'drink up' when clearly I'm trying to get healthy.
- Don't talk to my husband about it when I'm not around – if you're worried about me, talk to me.
- Don't say 'you poor thing' – we hate that!

And lastly …

- Yes please pick up my child or make us dinner while we're going through IVF – thank you!
- Please be patient with me, sometimes I'll need to tell all, sometimes I won't want to say a word about it.

'When I explained to a friend I had what I thought were early pregnancy signs but I had a negative test result she said, 'It's all in your head, you want to be pregnant so badly your brain is making you think you are.' I burst into tears.' **Karen, 38**

PS: Good friends will want to be there for you. You might just have to help them to help you.

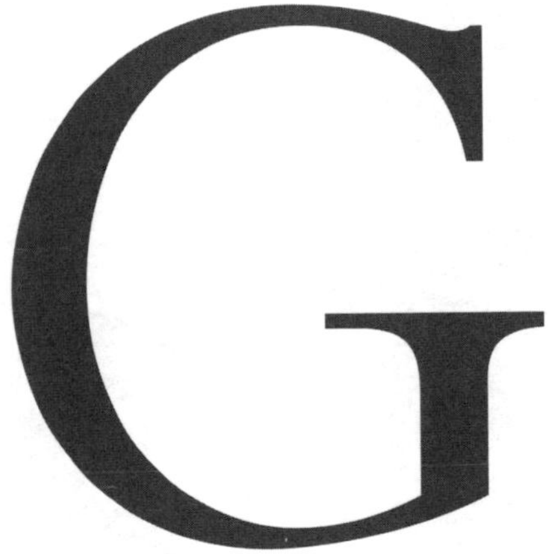

G is for getting on with tests and treatment

So you've been at it for six months straight, swinging your legs over your head after sex trying to steer your husband's sperm into your uterus like a fleshy pinball machine, and nothing? It might be time to get some basic tests done. If you're concerned, you should go and see your GP, especially

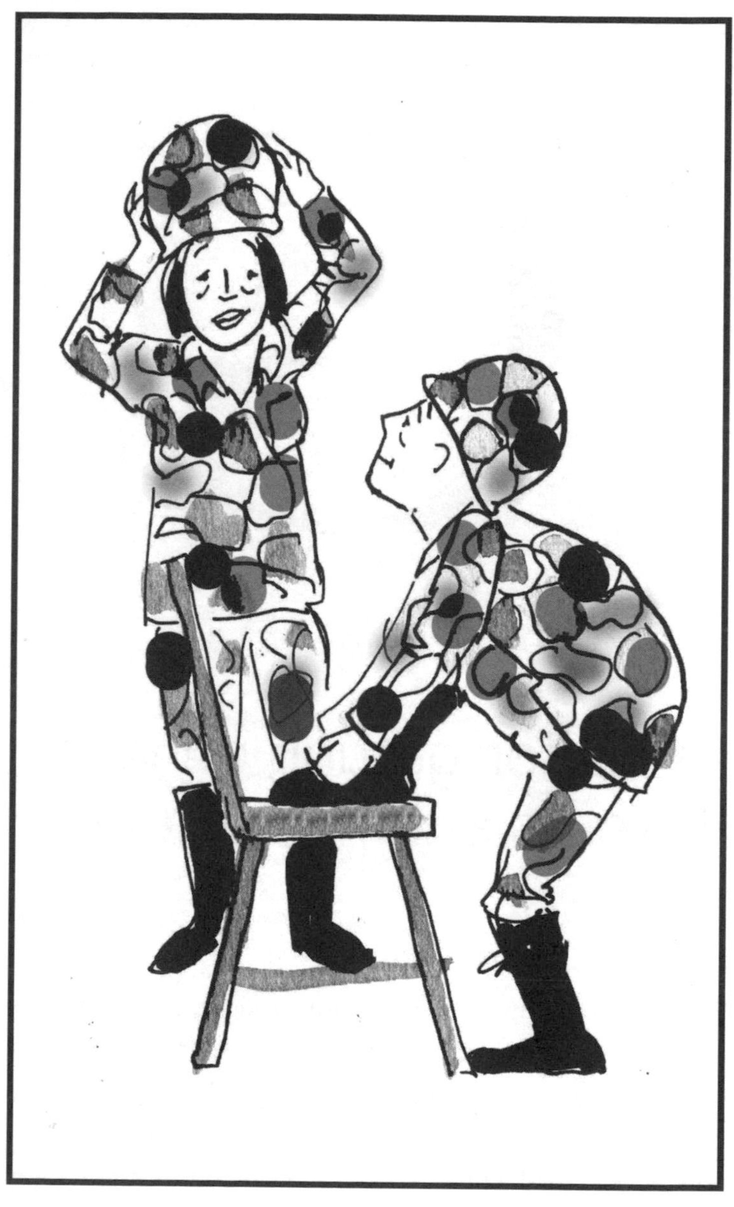

if you think medical history might play a part. They might send you for tests straight away, or suggest some lifestyle changes. After one year of trying, you will probably be sent for tests. Don't leave it any longer before visiting your GP. It can take a few months to get in to see a busy specialist so if you do want some basic tests done, then make the appointment now. You can always cancel it when you get pregnant *this* month. But for now …

When to go for tests

It's time to start going for tests when:

- you just want to know that everything is okay
- you don't want to waste any time wondering what might not be okay
- you have a sense something might be a bit off
- you know in your heart things are fine but you want the reassurance so you can get on with enjoying baby-making.

Getting tested does not commit you to any sort of treatment. If you have a few tests it doesn't mean you'll be injecting yourself for IVF next week. Not at all. Tests are reassuring. If you're in your mid-thirties, it just makes sense to check things out. To see if you have any endometriosis, for example, or any scarring in your fallopian tubes or just to see if your new partner's gizz is as impressive as his snuggling skills. The longer you are TTC the more you'll want answers – fast. So many problems with fertility are small and can be dealt with pretty easily. Waiting and wondering can add extra pressure. You start thinking 'Is it me? Is it you? Have we left this too late? What if it's something terrible? What if there aren't any eggs left? How expensive is treatment anyway?' Arrgh! Just take a deep breath and go for some reassuring tests – together.

> 'Basic tests are so simple and non-invasive. We'll see if there's sperm and if you're ovulating. A lot of people get basic tests early just so they don't have to worry.' **IVF specialist, Dr Bill Watkins**

Step 1

Go see your GP. Your doctor will ask questions about issues that may have a bearing on fertility such as if you have diabetes, any sexually transmitted diseases or any thyroid problems. She'll also want to know what medication you might be taking. Other questions may concern your sex life, the frequency of intercourse and the reproductive histories of your parents and siblings (how many babies they've had – not their sex life!). You'll also be asked if you've ever been pregnant and if it ended in a termination, miscarriage or, in fact, a baby. Don't be ashamed or embarrassed by your past. We all have one … grisly bits and all.

Step 2

A physical exam. Both of you will undergo a general physical exam that may include a smear test for you (knees up!).

Step 3

Semen analysis. Depending on your age, how long you have been trying or how keen you are for the tests, the next step – testing the sperm – happens at a fertility clinic. Your GP will give you a referral to see a fertility specialist. A low sperm count or poor sperm quality is behind between 30 and 40 per cent of infertility cases, so guys, it's time to step up (but I'm sure you can do it sitting down too). To do the test, the guy collects the sperm in a sterile container. He can do it at home but preferably at a fertility clinic. If he does it at home he'll have to hand it over at the fertility clinic within 40 minutes of 'depositing it' in the cup, so why put extra pressure on yourself? He'll also have to abstain from 'releasing' any sperm in the 48 hours prior – or thereabouts.

The sperm are checked for numbers, shape and motility. The seminal fluid is also checked for infection. Normal sperm motility should be greater than 50 per cent and sperm count should be above 15 million per ml. He shouldn't worry if it wasn't his 'best shot' or he spilled some trying to aim for the cup. Just getting as much as you can in there is fine. There's no rush and you can join him in there if you like, although most guys apparently do best on their own with the help of the kindly gals in the porno mags.

PS: Guys, the nurses are not judging you on how long it took you to whip up a 'sample' in the special room. Believe it or not, to them you're just a man with a little cup and a big sheepish grin.

Step 4

Hormone screening. Your blood and/or urine will be tested to check the levels of hormones needed for ovulation and implantation.

Step 5

Ultrasound. This is where sound waves are used to examine inside your uterus. This is an internal ultrasound, not an external one like those performed when pregnant. I loved meeting my uterus for the first time – fascinating stuff! Plus, I was a bit worried it may have skipped town during my Who-Needs-A-Uterus-Anyway single days. During the exam, a wand-shaped transducer is inserted into the vagina and images appear on a nearby monitor. Your practitioner will then take you on a guided tour of your ovaries, the uterus and follicles that hold the eggs before ovulation. Fibroid tumours and ovarian cysts can be detected in this test.

Step 6

Checking the grisly bits. Okay, so your fertility specialist may need to go a little deeper into your bits to check things out. You may need:

Hysterosalpinogram (HSG): This is an X-ray procedure where a special dye is injected through the cervix into the fallopian tubes to check whether passages are open or blocked. Most women say this one is uncomfortable (but not unbearable) and some cramping goes on.

Laparoscopy: This is a surgical procedure where a narrow fibre optic telescope is inserted through a tiny incision near your belly button. It allows your doctor to examine the uterus, fallopian tubes and ovaries, and to look for signs of endometriosis or pelvic adhesions. The procedure is done under general anesthesia in day surgery and you'll need to take about a week off work for post-operative rest and recovery. I had a laparoscopy and took a week off work to be waited on by Ben and read books (not fertility websites!). And the tiny little scar below my belly button disappeared in no time.

Of course, you probably won't rush into a fertility clinic and book in for a laparoscopy the following week. It's a systematic thing – one step at a time and lots of information is available along the way.

It's definitely a tense time waiting for test results but if you go into the experience supporting each other – no matter what the tests show – then you'll get through it just fine.

As I've said, tests can be reassuring. If everything is normal you can go back to happily swinging your legs over your head until you lose circulation in your feet.

Here are the two biggies on what *might* be wrong.

Polycystic ovarian syndrome (PCOS)

This is estimated to affect 5–10 per cent of women in the West. The term 'polycystic ovaries' means the ovaries contain lots of tiny cysts just beneath the surface of the ovaries. The cysts are due to hormonal imbalance and may not cause any problems at all. Or, some women develop additional symptoms such as irregular or absent periods, recurrent miscarriage and weight problems. The symptoms are triggered by an imbalance of sex hormones such as a high production of the androgen testosterone. Insulin is also a factor. Weight management and exercise will play an important role in treatment. Medication can also be taken to balance the hormones.

Endometriosis

Endometriosis is where the cells lining the inside of the uterus (the endometrium) establish themselves on the outside of the uterus in the pelvic area, the fallopian tubes, the ovaries, bladder or bowel (they get around!). Some symptoms include pain during sex, pain between periods, irregular bleeding and fatigue. Endometriosis can be detected via a laparoscopy and a surgeon can remove the cells from the affected areas.

It can also be treated with medication to control the hormones stimulating the symptoms. Women with endometriosis do go on to have babies – I have lots of TTC friends who've had 'endo'. Several got pregnant the very next month after the endo was removed.

It's not me, it's you: fertility problems in men

Some of the fertility problems found in men include:

- testicular disease
- obstructions (blocks in the tubes carrying sperm)
- hormonal problems
- medications that reduce fertility
- varicoceles (enlarged, or varicose, spermatic veins in the scrotum)
- trauma to the genital area
- sperm problems
- problems with ejaculation or erection
- environmental toxins and radiation.

That all sounds a bit scary (maybe don't show your partner the above) but most problems can be detected by a bit of prodding, poking and further testing by your fertility specialist.

So what *exactly* happens when they test sperm? Do a bunch of scientist guys sit around a table scoffing at your man's specimen, speculating how many times he's been kicked in the 'region'? It's a whole lot more scientific than that. So here's a run-down of what they test for during a basic sperm test …

- **Sperm count:** This is the total number of sperm in the whole sample (asuming he hasn't missed the pot – if he has, don't worry, it happens, and it's worth mentioning to the lab). A 'normal' sperm count is anything above 15 million per ml; the average sperm count in the west is 60 million per ml.
- **Motlility:** Around 60 per cent of sperm should be moving – the immobile ones can get in the way but are usually left behind. It's worth knowing that if the count is high and the motility low the overall sample can still be good.
- **Morphology:** This is the test for the good-looking sperm. They need the basics of a head and a tail ... There are other things they'll look for, but general good looks (and potential function) are the key to understanding morphology.
- **Volume:** This can be between 1.5ml and 6.5ml per sample. If you have seen a sample in a pot you will know it looks small – but don't be fooled and do your maths – a 3ml sample with 60 million per ml totals 180 million sperm.

There are lots of treatment options available for sperm. They include drug therapy to overcome hormone imbalance, artificial insemination (AI), surgery to correct varicoceles or to treat a blockage.

Unexplained infertility – what the *#$#?!

Unexplained infertility, as it's officially known, reportedly affects 20 per cent of all infertile couples. It's when fertility testing doesn't show up any physical problems but a pregnancy just doesn't happen – no matter how many times you kiss butt with the Baby Gods. A fertility specialist might simply put your case in the 'too hard' basket. When Ben and I were diagnosed with unexplained infertility we were told it could be 'psychological' or 'emotional'. More likely, just something small that they weren't picking up in their tests.

I used to drive myself crazy scouring Internet sites on what *might* be wrong. I'm sure I consumed so much information on infertility it made me infertile. So, instead of listing what *could* be wrong if you fall into this category, let's look at what needs to happen to ensure a healthy conception.

Timeline of a healthy conception

- The hormones that stimulate egg development are made in the brain and pituitary gland and then released properly.
- The egg is of good quality and chromosomally normal.
- The brain releases a surge of the LH hormone to stimulate final maturation of the egg.
- The follicle ruptures and releases follicular fluid and the egg.

- The fallopian tube picks up the egg.
- The sperm reaches the egg in the fallopian tube.
- The sperm penetrates the cumulus cells around the egg and releases its DNA (23 chromosomes) into the egg.
- The fertilised egg divides and the early embryo continues to divide.
- The fallopian tube will 'wave' the embryo into the uterus in three days and the embryo will develop into a blastocyst.
- The blastocyst hatches.
- Once hatched the blastocyct attaches to the uterine wall and implants.

So, sometimes in unexplained infertility something along this timeline is a bit out. Maybe you're not producing enough of the right hormones or the sperm doesn't have 'egg cracking' capabilities. There are a lot of treatment options. There are even more little things you can do outside a fertility clinic that will make a real difference to boosting your fertility and might just be the answer. Here are a few ideas for your next cycle.

When things aren't working but nothing is wrong

- Try acupuncture.
- Overhaul your lifestyle and load up on fertility super foods (see 'H is for healthy living').
- Ask yourself how stressed you are.
- Try using an ovulation predictor kit (OPK) this month.

- Just have sex every second day through your whole cycle.
- Try sperm-friendly lubricants such as PreSeed.
- Get more sleep.
- Learn a few key points in reflexology and start massaging each other's feet.
- Get your man on a zinc supplement.
- Consider a round of intrauterine insemination (IUI).

Choices, choices

It's likely that the first step after seeing your GP will be some basic investigations .... bloods, sperm test, medical history and lifestyle check. The next step is usually a trip to the local fertility clinic where you will be assesed and, if possible, given a diagnosis. Getting your results may take time, so try and be patient.

At this point treatment options are discussed and a plan of care established. There is a good choice of treatments available in most clinics. To find out what's available to you locally, go to the Human Fertility & Embryology Authority website (www.hfea.gov.uk) where you will find your local clinics and the services they offer. I've given you the basic treatments below; there are other, more complicated, treaments available, but these are usually recommended for specific reasons, e.g. genetic problems.

- **Drugs:** You may be offered drugs which improve ovulation, improve your menstrual cycle (periods) or balance hormones ... the list is vast. Simple drugs treatments involve taking a few tablets at the begining of a cycle which gives you a super-charged ovulation (which you'd use a OPK to detect). If after a few cycles of this you've not concieved, they may change the drugs to more powerful injections. It may be that IUI is used alongside the drugs.

- **IUI (intrauterine insemination):** Your man will have to produce a sample from which his best sperm are selected and inserted via a fine tube into the womb. The timing is usually just after ovulation so the two can conveniently meet in the fallopian tubes. The pluses are it's fairly non-invasive, there aren't any injections (unless you have one injection to help trigger ovulation) and it's not as expensive as IVF. The down side is you have be to extremely savvy in the timing to get the sperm into the right spot right on ovulation. Lots of couples try a few rounds of IUI before embarking on IVF. Does it work? Yes. I've read lots of cases of it working the very first time! It didn't work for us but I blame a very slow cycle that month (I think I ovulated on day 26!) because of lots of stress. Does it hurt? No, it's just a little uncomfortable.
- **Donor sperm:** Any donor sperm is screened and selected. The donor goes through a rigourous screening process. Donor sperm can be used in IVF or IUI.

- **Surgery:** Surgery is only needed if there are significant abnormalities. They may include vaginal, cervical, uterine or ovarian abnormalities, or blocked uterine tubes.

PS: Try to remember your husband's date of birth when they bring out the sperm sample during IUI. They'll ask you a few security questions about your man to make sure they have the right sample for the job (imagine messing that up!) and I totally forgot Ben's birth date. Mind you, at his first semen analysis test Ben forgot the name of our doctor and sat in the sperm deposit room for 20 minutes trying to call me at my work to ask me. He was worried the nurses were thinking he had actual problems in there ...

IVF

Ever since the first 'test-tube baby' Louise Brown was born in 1978 women have been turning to IVF to help create miracles they just can't achieve on their own (no matter how many times they bribe the Baby Gods). Put very simply, IVF is the joining of an egg and sperm in the lab (*in vitro*). The fertilised egg is placed back in the woman's uterus and everything happens pretty much as it would normally from there (she crosses her fingers – and legs – and drives herself crazy during the Two Week Wait to see if she is pregnant).

The technical stuff ...

A typical IVF cycle

A cycle of IVF treatment typically follows these steps:

1. Preparation for stimulated cycle.
2. Egg pick up and semen collection.
3. Laboratory grows embryos.
4. Embryo transfer, embryo freezing and storage.
5. Pregnancy test.

Let's look at each of these steps in detail.

1. Preparation for stimulated cycle

The ovaries are stimulated with medications known as gonadotropins (hormones). They are injected into the fatty tissue underneath the skin every day for a period of eight to 14 days. Stimulated cycles also use additional medications through other injections or nasal sprays at different times in the cycle. The treatment is monitored with vaginal ultrasound scanning and blood tests.

2. Egg pick up and semen collection

This is the surgical collection of eggs from the ovaries (known as harvesting). The egg pick up is performed in the operating theatre with either light sedation or general anesthetic. An internal ultrasound is performed via the vagina to locate the ovaries. A needle is then passed through the top of the vagina into each ovary and the fluid and the eggs are retrieved from the follicles. The procedure generally takes about 15–30 minutes and hospital discharge is usually a few hours later.

A semen sample is also collected at this stage in preparation for fertilisation of the eggs. Men are advised to save up sperm (i.e. don't ejaculate) for 48 hours in preparation. The 'deposit' can be made at the IVF clinic on the day of egg pick up.

3. Laboratory grows embryos

After pick up and sperm collection, the eggs and sperm are prepared for fertilisation either through IVF (whereby and egg and sperm are mixed together) or ICSI (a microinjection where a single sperm is injected into the centre of an egg for fertilisation to occur). The 'mixtures' are then placed in a secure, warm environment and monitored at controlled times to check on development. If fertilisation is successful, the process continues.

4. Embryo transfer, embryo freezing and storage

Embryo transfer usually happens two days after egg pick up. The procedure only takes a few minutes. Usually no anesthetic is required for transfer and any discomfort is minor – similar to a smear test. The cervix is cleansed with a solution to remove old blood and mucus. The embryos are placed in a fine catheter tube, passed through the cervix via the cervical canal and deposited at the top of the uterus. (Some 'leaking' may be experienced afterwards but that's just the cleansing solution. The embryo is securely in the uterus and can't 'leak out'.)

Most fertility specialists will recommend just one embryo at a time is transferred but it's your decision; you might want to transfer two and cross your fingers one takes or you end up with healthy fraternal twins! Women over 40 tend to have 3 embryos transferred.

Freezing: One or two embryos are chosen for transfer while the remaining suitable embryos can be frozen, usually for an additional charge. They can then be used for transfer in subsequent cycles. Many women going through IVF affectionately call such embryos their 'frosties'. The embryos are placed in a protective medium and loaded into a straw with the patient's details. They are frozen gradually to -150°C. They are then transferred to a liquid nitrogen storage tank that holds the temperature at -196°C.

5. Pregnancy test

The result probably won't be tested by your fertility specialist any earlier than 16 days after transfer (this is the Two Week Wait). A test detects the level of human chorionic gonadotropin (HCG). You can test earlier at home if you'd like to (of course!). A blood test will be carried out by your fertility specialist after 16 days whether you have already started your period or not. A little blood may still mean you are pregnant.

And now to the emotional stuff ....

Stress

IVF is without doubt one of the most stressful infertility treatments. But you can alleviate the stress by seeking out, through your clinic or hospital, an IVF counsellor at the very start of the journey, securing close family support to take care of you and any other children you may have, getting lots of rest, good food and gentle, regular exercise.

Sticking together

I hear so many stories of couples going through IVF and coming out the other end so much closer for the experience. You are joined in your mission both physically (especially if he's helping with injections or it's a sperm thing) and emotionally. You'll cry together, you'll pray together, you'll laugh at silly things that only you as a couple will find funny in the process together, you'll be mad, you'll make up, you'll be there for each other at the end of the cycle. You'll never look back from a life-changing event together like IVF.

Psychologist and IVF counsellor Lynne Quayle says it's important to be gentle with each other, to acknowledge each other's feelings (even though you're the one taking all the injections). Tell him what you need even if it's just a cuddle on the couch every night. Guys aren't mind readers (no matter how loudly we sigh at them). You have to gently spell things out along the way. And keep asking him questions too. Keep cuddling, keep talking and keep forgiving each other for not being perfect.

'It needs to be a team effort all the way with your partner, sharing dreams, fears and disappointments with honesty and trust. While lots of sharing will be IVF-related, make sure it's not only about that. Remember all of the other things on which your bond is based.'

Psychologist and IVF counsellor, Lynne Quayle

Telling people you're trying IVF

Do you tell people what you're going through? This is tricky. Here are some of the pros for telling them:

- You won't get annoying 'Are you trying for a baby?' questions from people who know.
- If anything goes wrong (such as an ectopic pregnancy or miscarriage) you'll have immediate support and the loss will be acknowledged.
- If you need to take time off work, your boss will be more understanding if he or she knows that you're going through IVF.
- Keeping such a big secret may add to the stress.
- You may need the practical day-to-day help of your family if you already have a child.

'Some women need to talk, others just want to knuckle down and get on with it.'

IVF specialist, Dr Bill Watkins

And here are some of the cons:

- People will inevitably ask insensitive questions you may not want to answer.
- You might not tell people you're TTC naturally; why give up that privacy when you're going through IVF?
- If you told a family member, could you really trust that they wouldn't blab to their friends or other family members?
- If you did have an ectopic pregnancy or miscarriage, you might not want to share your grief with anyone but your partner.
- Knowing people are talking about your private life may add to the pressure.

> 'When you get through IVF you know you can get through anything.' **Emma, 34**

It's a very personal decision. A good TTC friend of mine had this advice: Yes, tell the people closest to you that you are going through IVF for the support and the help with everyday life along the way (especially if you already have a small child). But don't tell them how many rounds you are planning to have or where you are in the cycle. Staying vague reduces the amount of questions (they'll get the hint!) but having them know means you have their support. Plus, if one round doesn't work but you don't want the added pressure and disappointment felt by your family and close friends, don't tell them you are going for another round and just do it secretly. You can tell them later – when you're expecting twins.

> 'Some people feel they have entered a parallel universe. It's easy to forget or ignore what was normal life including the pre-IVF you. It's a stronger stance to have a foot in each universe, drawing on the strengths from each. Maintaining a social life, maintaining friendships and a sense of belonging and distraction, affirms you as an individual and as a couple. The foot in the IVF world is where you are discovering new things about yourself. Did you know you could feel so emotional and still survive? Did you think it was possible that you would be tempted to avoid your best friend just because she is pregnant? IVF hopefully provides an opportunity for self-development rather than self-abandonment. Whether you succeed in IVF or not, you still want a healthy, functioning you at the end of it.' **Psychologist and IVF counsellor, Lynne Quayle**

Keeping everyday life going

They don't call IVF a roller-coaster just because there are obvious ups and downs. Maybe it's because it goes fast then painfully slow in the Two Week Wait and you never know just how scared and excited you were until you reach the very end. With most of us already leading such busy lives, keeping up with the demands of IVF can place unbearable pressure on couples. If things are getting on top of you, it might be an idea to make a list of all your commitments and start striking off the ones that you can get out of. It's important to say no to people and give yourself a break. Scale down your life/work commitments as much as you can so the focus is on you, the treatment, your partner, staying well and positive and turning up to work on time, unless you can take a few weeks off here and there.

> 'The injections, blood tests, ultrasounds, progesterone creams were all just a mechanical process for me and didn't really phase me but it was the daily ups and downs that really knocked me about. On any given day I was either filled with so much hope or so much hopelessness.' **Eliza, 34**

Here are a few ways to make everyday life easier:

- Know where you'll be each day for injection time.
- Know who will be giving your injection and that they are organised to be there too. Unless, of course, you are giving yourself the injections.
- Give yourself plenty of time to calm down and rest before and after injections.
- Delegate a few tasks at work to others – without any guilt!
- Make a double batch of dinner and freeze it for later in the week.

- Work regular exercise into your everyday routine – get off the bus a few stops early and walk the rest of the way to work.
- Don't schedule in social events you really don't want to go to.
- Say no.
- Organise for your other child or children to be picked up from nursery for you so you can get to doctor's appointments.
- Don't miss appointments with your IVF counsellor – they are a priority.
- Have a plan with your partner regarding who will cook and who will clean each week – so there aren't any arguments.
- Make time to rest (that means scheduling in time for yourself as you would a business meeting or date with friends – no breaking appointments!).

'When I was in IVF I had a bath ritual every day. I would lather up in my favourite soap and then I'd try to imagine all my fears and anxiety going down the drain. It was one small way of keeping me sane until we got pregnant in the third cycle.' **Lynne, 39**

Your support team

So you've let a few people know you're in IVF. Just how do you let them help you? Give them roles to play out so it's clear what's expected of them and what you need (which may change).

Here are some suggestions of things to say:

'I just need you to distract me.'

'I just need a shoulder to cry on.'

'Today I need a good laugh.'

'I need you to tell me I'm an okay person.'

'It's only a little step forward but today I need to celebrate.'

'I need you to cheer up my husband – take him out for a beer.'

'Please just be the one who reminds me to pick up the dry cleaning.'

> 'The most important support person is you. Everyone else is a bonus. How can you support yourself? Be kind to yourself, be tolerant of that full range of emotions you are going to experience, be assertive and continue to shore up your emotional resilience.'
>
> **Psychologist and IVF counsellor, Lynne Quayle**

Staying positive

I read so many posts by women in online TTC forums asking just *how* they can stay positive when IVF fails, when they miscarry, when they're feeling so scared and alone they don't know what to do any more. Well, you won't hear 'buck up' and 'you're not alone' here. This is your experience and you and only you are experiencing it in your own way. It can all feel incredibly lonely, no matter how big your support team is. Just because women have been here before does not make you weak or not as strong as those who have it 'worse' than you. Your experience is your experience.

IVF counsellor and psychologist Lynne Quayle advises you should give yourself permission to be upset and angry. Cry, get it all out of your body, make time to grieve, and grieve some more. Don't rush through your feelings or bottle them up and try to 'cope better' next time. Keep watch on yourself. Are you more than unhappy? Go see someone. It doesn't mean you're not coping – the opposite! People who seek out help *are* coping by getting help when they need it. Being positive or optimistic might be a choice we make every day, just as we can choose to be happy. You might want to tell yourself each morning, 'Today I am *choosing* to be optimistic'. Tomorrow you can be negative and miserable (you won't want to be!) but just for today, choose to be optimistic and see how you go.

Meanwhile, surround yourself with the people who enrich your life and, most of all, make you smile. Make time for the people and the little occasions that make you happy.

Simple things are the best – a bath with your partner, a good long phone chat with an old mate overseas, walking your dog, baking a chocolate cake with your niece and then eating it with her in a tea party for two. Try to keep things simple, unhurried, as stress-free as possible. Most of all, no matter what, *refuse to be busy*. Plan early on how you would best like to cope. Talk it over with your partner and, remember, plans can change.

> ‘The first cycle is full of excitement and anticipation. If not successful the next few times, however, stress can increase and patients usually revert to old coping strategies like anger, blaming, helplessness or conversely, positive thinking. Some will moderate their emotions by not raising their hopes up, hoping this will make it easier to handle disappointment. A good tip is to work out early in the process what works best for you.’
>
> **Psychologist and IVF counsellor, Lynne Quayle**

For relatives and friends, what *not* to say to someone in IVF

‘I know how you feel.’

‘You poor thing.’

‘It’s probably for the best.’

‘Could you have tried harder?’

‘Could the doctors have messed it up?’

‘Is it getting expensive?’

‘Science can’t beat nature.’

'Do you get the money back when it doesn't work?'
'At what age do they just stop trying?'

Try not to:

- ask too many questions
- forget your role
- skim over the importance of loss should there be a miscarriage
- tell her to 'buck up' for next time without letting her grieve
- tiptoe around her
- treat her like an infertile freak
- be upset when she doesn't turn up to events with babies involved.

' It's hard being a support person – even when you've gone through IVF yourself! I was a support person for my sister and she changed her mind almost every day on what she wanted from me. It was exhausting trying to read her emotions and do the right thing. I just had to roll with it and try to keep up – but we all got through it. You just do. ' **Deb, 34**

PS: Everyone has tough stuff they go through in life. Congratulate yourself every day for getting through fertility tests and treatment – you're amazing!

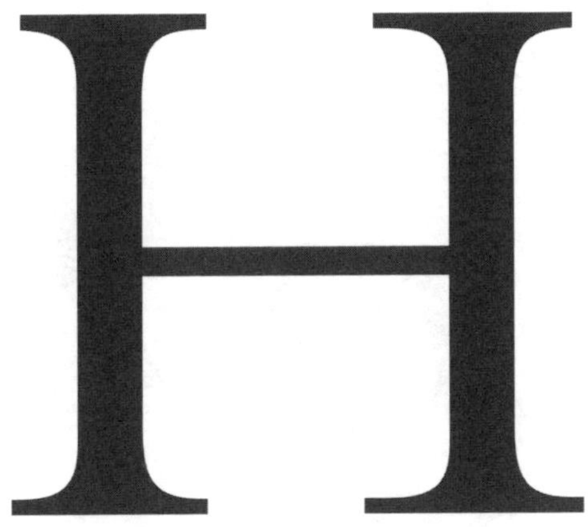

H is for healthy living

We know, we *know*! It's time to spruce up the sperm, get ourselves in tip-top fertility-friendly shape and stop drinking four glasses of chardonnay on a Friday night (blah, blah). But *how* healthy do we have to be? That was always the question I was asking myself when we were TTC. How healthy is healthy?

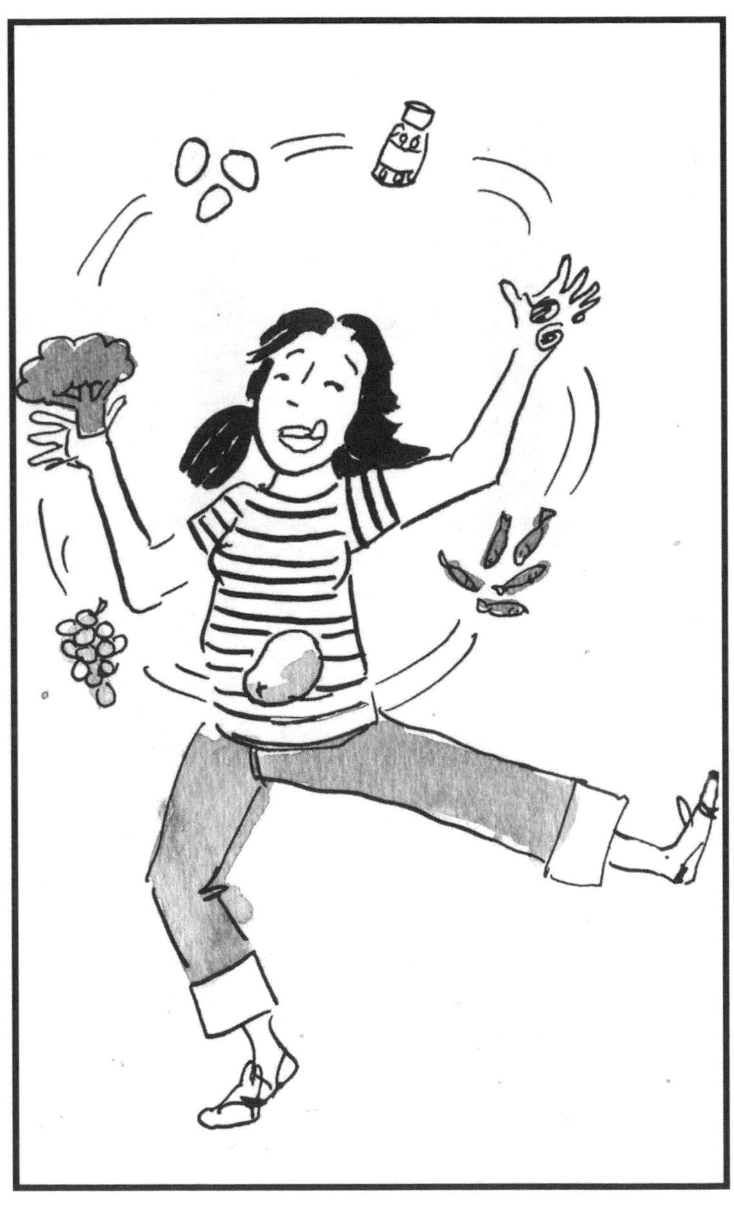

If you read some books out there on baby-making, living the simple life and eating organics is the only way to conceive a child. But who on earth can stop using their mobile phone, move to the country, stay away from power lines, never drink wine and only eat organics? Well, not many of us. Believe me, I put it to my husband Ben and he nearly choked on his chicken nuggets and chips.

Quick quiz: How fertility-friendly is your lifestyle?

1. Do you or your partner lose count of the drinks you have at parties?
2. Do you or your partner ever smoke cigarettes or weed?
3. Do you forget to eat two pieces of fruit and five portions of vegetables a day?
4. Are you overweight? Underweight?
5. Do you or your partner stress a lot?
6. Do you fail to get a good walk in most days?
7. Do you rarely drink a total of 2 litres of water a day?
8. Is this list starting to tick you off?

If you answered 'yes' to most of the above then yep, you might be a bit of a maggot (hey, aren't we all!). If you answered 'no' to most then you're already on track – break out the carrot sticks! If you're somewhere in between then sprucing up your lifestyle will be a walk in the park (okay, maybe a jog).

Let's start with the basics, beginning today.

Fertility booster plan – starting *now*

- Eat more berries or citrus fruits such as oranges and grapefruit (vitamin C will help boost sluggish sperm).
- Eat wholegrain food such as wholegrain bread (with lots of seeds in it), breakfast cereal and oats (wholegrain rolled oats – not 'quick oats' – are a TTC super food).
- Drink 2 litres of water – every day (flush out those toxins).
- Top up your iron with some lean red meat.
- Eat low-fat cheese, yoghurt and milk (keep your weight in a healthy range).
- Start drinking fertility-friendly herbal tea like ginger and peppermint instead of regular teas and coffee or, even better, drink lots of warm water with a wedge of lemon in it. (Cut right down on caffeine.)

Shake that booty

Along with eating fertility super foods and upping your Zen, exercising is the best way to get your body baby-ready in no time. Exercise oxygenates the body and increases the blood flow in order to supply your reproductive organs with essential oxygen. Walking is the easiest way to kick-start any exercise program so, if you're just dusting off your Nikes, start with a 20-minute walk three days the first week. If you're feeling energised, make it half an hour's walk every second day the next week and gradually work up to an hour's walk every day. Add some gentle stretching before your walk and especially afterwards. Walking to work is also a great way to exercise without feeling like you're working too hard at it, so maybe get off the bus a few stops early or resist taking the car. If you already have kids, walk to your local park and join in with their play. Don't go too hard and fast when you're starting a new exercise routine during TTC as strenuous exercise more than three times a week may inhibit your chances of conceiving. Start out gently and work on your fitness gradually by making it fun, something to look forward to which fits in easily with your lifestyle and something which does not call for lycra . . .

The Bump & Grind exercise plan

- Go for a 20-minute walk three days the first week.
- Do lots of stretching before and especially after your walk.
- Gradually increase your walk times to half an hour every second day the next week and then an hour every day (take a few weeks to get there!).
- Make exercise fun – meet with a girlfriend for evening walks, go to an aerobics class at your

gym or drag your man to a salsa dance class at a local dance studio.

- Rent or buy a Pilates DVD to do in the comfort of your lounge room (start with a beginners programme).
- Try swimming laps at your local pool or go to a yoga class at your gym or local yoga centre – both will relax you, especially during the Two Week Wait.
- Join a gym and have a personal trainer show you exactly what to do to lose weight, tone up and have your body baby-ready in no time (remember, don't go too hard too fast). If you don't feel like telling the trainer you're trying to get fit to get pregnant just say you want to lose weight (but not too much too soon) and tone up, without lifting super-heavy weights. Even if you only join a gym to walk for 30 minutes on a treadmill during your lunch hour it will bring enormous benefits to your reproductive health. You don't have to become a gym junkie or break out the bicycle pants (phew).
- Have sweaty sex! Did you know an hour of 'vigorous' sex burns up to 300 calories?

PS: The only time really vigorous exercise isn't recommended when you're TTC is during the Two Week Wait when it's important to rest your body (and calm your mind) so give yourself

permission to go slow. Keep up your daily walks of course and enjoy dancing or swimming if it makes you feel good. Just don't push yourself to go to a 'pump' or 'core' class.

> 'With better lifestyle choices, there won't be so many women needing IVF and those who we do see will have much better results. We've had a lot of big milestones in IVF since it began and, really, lifestyle and fertility preservation now is the main issue.' **IVF specialist, Dr Bill Watkins**

Out with the bad, in with the good

When aiming to improve your health and therefore your fertility, you'll need to not only start eating healthier foods but also cut down on some unhealthy choices. Let's start with what you shouldn't be eating. Chuck out all the fertility-unfriendly food in your kitchen, such as the things listed below.

- Chips and any other salty, processed snack food. Salt has been blamed for impaired ovulation and increased blood pressure.
- Anything with aspartame (an artificial sweetener) in it. You'll find it in diet products such as soft drinks, diet yoghurts and sugar substitutes. Aspartame is linked with depression, weight gain, dizziness, palpitations, infertility and miscarriage (nasty stuff!). Read the packaging carefully.
- Fried foods. Too much saturated fat can contribute to

insulin resistance, endometriosis and PCOS. You can still have fries with that – bake your spuds in the oven in a little olive oil and sprinkle on some sea salt instead of the junky version.

The top 10 fertility super foods

1. Eggs. The humble egg provides vitamins A, B1, B2, B5 and B6, as well as iron, manganese and zinc *and* amino acids vital in sperm and egg production (*your* eggs, that is).

2. Porridge. Wholegrain rolled oats are a magical fertility super food. They release energy slowly as they are low GI and help regulate sugar levels and hormone production. Oats have long been considered a sexual energiser for horses *and* men, thus the phrase 'sowing your wild oats'. Giddee up!

3. Dates. These were considered a powerful aphrodisiac back in ancient times. They are a good source of iron and potassium for better general reproductive health. They are yummy eaten with chopped apple or chopped and tossed over your porridge.

4. Wheatgerm. It may taste like shaved cardboard but wheatgerm is chockers with magical vitamin E, zinc, selenium and B vitamins. It's worth adding a spoonful or two to a smoothie or on top of your cereal with natural yoghurt and pectin-packed berries.

5. Mangoes. Loaded with vitamin C – essential for fertility – and antioxidants to help counter the shiraz you drank on Friday night.

6. Kale. Spinach or broccoli will do the trick here too. These greens provide folic acid which we all know reduces your chances of having a baby with neural tube damage. Broccoli will also give you vitamin B5 – important for embryo development – so go big on broccoli when you're TTC, just in case!

7. Weird little slippery fish. Sardines, mackerel, herring and tuna are full of selenium and essential fatty acids that are good for regulating your hormones.

8. Pumpkin seeds and sunflower seeds. Both contain plenty of zinc. Zinc is a TTC champion because it helps maintain a healthy menstrual cycle and increases sperm count. Throw seeds over your porridge or cereal or into rice dishes, or just eat a handful with dried apricots.

9. Brazil nuts. Rich in selenium. Grab a handful along with raw almonds. And go nuts.

10. Lentils. Pulses have lots of the fertility powerhouse zinc, they fill you up and are a good source of fibre. Plus they are cheap and are delicious in curries and soups.

High alkaline foods

A diet rich in alkaline foods (as opposed to acidic) is good for cervical mucus and general reproductive health. High alkaline foods include apples, asparagus, avocados, bamboo shoots, cabbage, cherries, cucumber, leeks, olives, onions, peaches and potatoes. A chunkier list of alkaline foods, as well as acidic foods to avoid, can be found in 'W is for Way of the Bunny Rabbit' (those bunnies *love* alkaline foods).

Zinc and vitamin C

These two are said to be the greatest boosters for sluggish sperm. Fill him up on fish, grains and seeds, kiwifruit, leafy greens and tomatoes. A good-quality zinc supplement is also great for sperm – get him to take a small slug of it on its own (not with a meal). You can buy zinc supplements at chemists or health food shops.

Putting it all together

Not in a salad, please! The trick is – don't diet. Fill up on as many super foods as you can and shake that booty a little harder every day but make sure you enjoy eating. Getting your body ready to have a baby should not be hard work (because TTC is hard enough). It should be fun, easy and inexpensive. You should *both* enjoy it. Most of all, do not stress too much about getting your new eating plan exactly right all the time. Allow yourself slip-ups without any guilt and just try to do better the next day. If you don't like lentils and can't face pumpkin seeds – don't go there. Make up for it with fertility super foods that you do like.

Everyday eating plan

Breakfast: Porridge topped with chopped dates and sunflower seeds.

Snack: Mango slices or an orange.

Lunch: Turkey wrap with lots of dark leafy greens.

Snack: Sliced up apple with a blob of brazil nut paste.

Dinner: Lentil and vegetable curry with a dollop of natural yoghurt, mango chutney and brown rice.
Snack: Fresh (or frozen) berries.

On another day:
Breakfast: Two boiled eggs on grainy bread with steamed spinach and tomatoes.
Snack: Handful of raw almonds and an apple.
Lunch: Chunky vegetable soup with chickpeas or lentils.
Snack: Natural yoghurt with kiwifruit and brazil nuts.
Dinner: Seared tuna fillet and a leafy green salad with boiled potatoes.
Snack: A couple of dates.

Sneaky instant fertility boosters:

- Throw a handful of toasted pumpkin seeds into a vegetable curry (nice and crunchy!).
- Spoon some wheatgerm over your morning oats.
- Chop up some dates and add them to cereal.
- Add a handful of chopped brazil nuts to rice dishes.
- Blend your berries into a smoothie.
- Add a boiled egg to your lunchbox and slice it up in a sandwich.
- Dip carrot sticks into brazil or almond nut paste.

Goodbye toxins

It's oh-so annoying that the things we love, like splurging on wine and choc-chip ice cream, are so damn bad for us.

There goes my Friday night! Alas, there's no denying a healthy lifestyle will dramatically improve your chances of getting pregnant. So why do we see so many women smoking and drinking with five little kids at their side? Because they're probably a lot younger than us, and simply, the Baby Gods *suck*. I have tried the Recklessly Unhealthy Who Cares Piss-up Diet to get pregnant and sadly, it didn't work, it just gave me a headache. Healthy living is the only way to go.

> 'Adopt a healthy lifestyle now and the quality of your egg and sperm will dramatically improve in a couple of months.' **Dr Anne Clark, Fertility Society of Australia chair**

Booze – the scary news

Alcohol consumption is associated with hypothalmic-pituitary-ovarian dysfunction resulting in amenorrhea (absence of menstruation), anovulation (lack of ovulation) and luteal phase defects (abnormal development of the endometrial lining). Plus, we all know that, should you get pregnant, drinking alcohol puts you and your baby at risk of miscarriage, pre-term birth and stillbirth.

In men, alcohol may result in abnormal liver function and a rise in oestrogen levels, which may interfere with sperm development and hormone levels. Alcohol is also a toxin that can kill off the sperm-generating cells in the testicle. Because sperm takes at least three months to develop you should try a semen analysis again after three or four months of not drinking to properly check out your sperm.

It's been recommended women have no more than three standard glasses of wine a week and don't save them all up to have in one night. For men, no more than two standard drinks a day. Just to be sure, though, lots of health experts say you should lose the booze completely when you're TTC.

Cigarettes

There are more than 4,000 active substances in cigarette smoke. At least 20 of them are known to be mutagens, capable of causing genetic damage. Men who smoke are more likely to have children with congenital abnormalities or a higher risk of developing health problems such as asthma. If you smoke, it can take up to two months longer for you to conceive than a non-smoking couple. Quitting helps immediately. Your chances are dramatically improved if you combine quitting smoking with quitting booze, taking the right supplements and getting to a healthy weight. Plus, there's no way you'd smoke when you *are* pregnant so to make things easier – quit now.

Quitting – TTC style

Quitting smoking is hard at the best of times. When you get your period and break out the commiseration vinos it can be near impossible not to sneak in a few rogue cigarettes. But as we know, it all ends badly with smoking and you know you'll regret it afterwards. Here are some TTC Quit Tips that might help. Starting today:

- Picture that little egg (soon to be your baby) inside your body – you don't want to choke it with smoke and nasty chemicals.
- Stay away from alcohol if that's a trigger to smoke – especially when you get your period.
- Scare yourself with stats if that works – did you know women who smoke reportedly age their ovaries by up to 10 years? Eeeks! A whole decade!
- Don't be too hard on yourself and just do better and better each day until you have quit.
- Congratulate yourself every time you resist a fag – it'll make you feel stronger and stronger.
- Get help – patches or gum still fill your system with nicotine, and thus help with cravings, but it's better than smoking. Use them to cut down and quit.
- Don't be around smokers.
- You're about to become a mum. You wouldn't smoke with your newborn baby nearby so quit now.

> 'There will be real improvements to egg quality the month before you ovulate if you quit now and a dramatic improvement in two months if you stay quit. Plus, if the man stops smoking, DNA damage of the sperm can be reduced dramatically in months to come.'
>
> **Dr Anne Clark, Fertility Society of Australia chair**

Marijuana

Marijuana causes changes to sperm mobility and can reduce sperm count, decreasing its effectiveness. It also decreases the volume of seminal fluid. Sperm from weed smokers is more likely to swim too fast too early, leading to burn-out before they reach the egg.

Women's fertility is also adversely affected by weed smoking. Marijuana increases prolactin, interfering with the menstrual cycle and ovulation. It also affects the placenta and could prevent implantation.

Caffeine

If you have more than 100mg of caffeine per day (equal to one espresso cup of coffee or two instant coffees, two cups of black tea or three cups of green tea) you can reportedly reduce your chances of conceiving by up to 50 per cent. Caffeine is also found in cola drinks, energy drinks and chocolate. Cut right down on coffee when you are TTC or, even better, join the chai latte set and ask that you have a liquid chai mix without any black tea in it – just spices.

The great weight debate

I was told by the Fertility Sisters that I should lose 1.5 stone before getting pregnant. *What now*?! It was one thing to get fit and lose the booze but drop 1.5 stone? I almost choked on my Pringles. But instead of getting depressed about it (who ate the last Kit Kat anyway?) I hauled my big butt to the gym and started walking an hour to work. I didn't lose anywhere near 1.5 stone before getting pregnant – more like half – but upping the exercise was a good way to rela– sorry, chill out during TTC anyway.

So how much weight does the weight debate hold in fertility anyway?

Big fat stats

- Infertility in obese and overweight women is primarily related to ovulatory dysfunction.
- Studies have shown that 30 to 47 per cent of obese women (that is, with a BMI over 30) have irregular menstrual cycles.
- Your body mass index (BMI) only has to be three points higher than the normal range (20–25) and you are three times less likely to be ovulating.

> 'The good news is women only need to lose a bit of weight, such as a stone, and 90 per cent of them will go back to normal ovulation.'
>
> **Dr Anne Clark, Fertility Society of Australia chair**

How to lose weight fast *and* stay baby ready and healthy

- Try not to diet for TTC – it can feel like too long and hard a road ahead and add to the pressure of TTC when it's already stressful enough! Lose weight for *you* (and your skinny jeans).
- Eat a good breakfast.
- Don't stop eating fertility super foods with good fats like nuts and seeds.
- Don't skip meals.
- Fill up on vegetable soup for lunch and/or dinner (make up a batch of it and freeze portions).
- Don't quit carbs (go for small servings of good carbs such as grainy bread).
- Snack on seeds and dried apricots instead of junk.
- Eat a small dinner.
- *Don't* eat diet products like yoghurt or drink diet soft drinks containing the artificial sweetener aspartame (bad for fertility).
- Add dark leafy greens to lunch and dinner.
- Avoid too much stress – reports say stress can add to weight problems.

- Drink lots and lots of warm water with fresh lemon in it (have a big jug on your desk and drink through the day).
- Get lots of sleep.
- Up your cardio workout.
- Have lots of sex – good cardio!

'I used to try and diet for TTC but it made me depressed. I wanted to lose the weight *now* but couldn't and every time I got my period I'd slip into bad habits. Eventually I stopped trying to diet and just get healthier – it worked. Plus, I think babies like a soft house – a little bit of padding here and there!' **Lynne, 39**

PS: A healthy mind and a happy heart are just as important as how many sunflower seeds you can chow down. See 'V is for visualisations and magical stuff'.

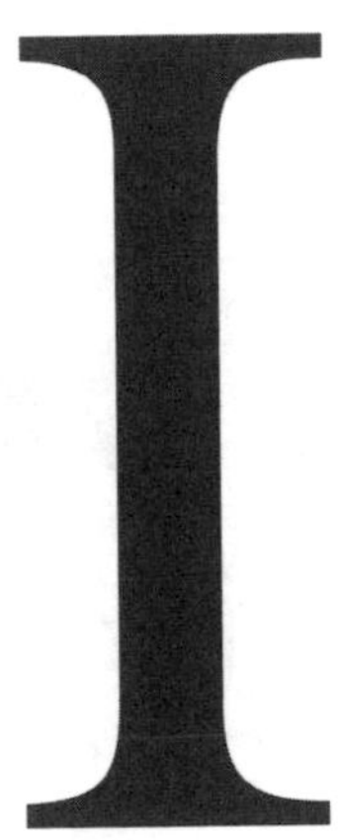

I is for Internet angels

You won't hear a woman who's trying to get pregnant answer 'How are you?' with 'I'm ovulating, darls!' or 'I'm on cycle day 17 so, you know, mental.'

And fair enough.

Most women keep their TTC efforts to themselves. We don't want to jinx our luck, we don't want a sympathetic

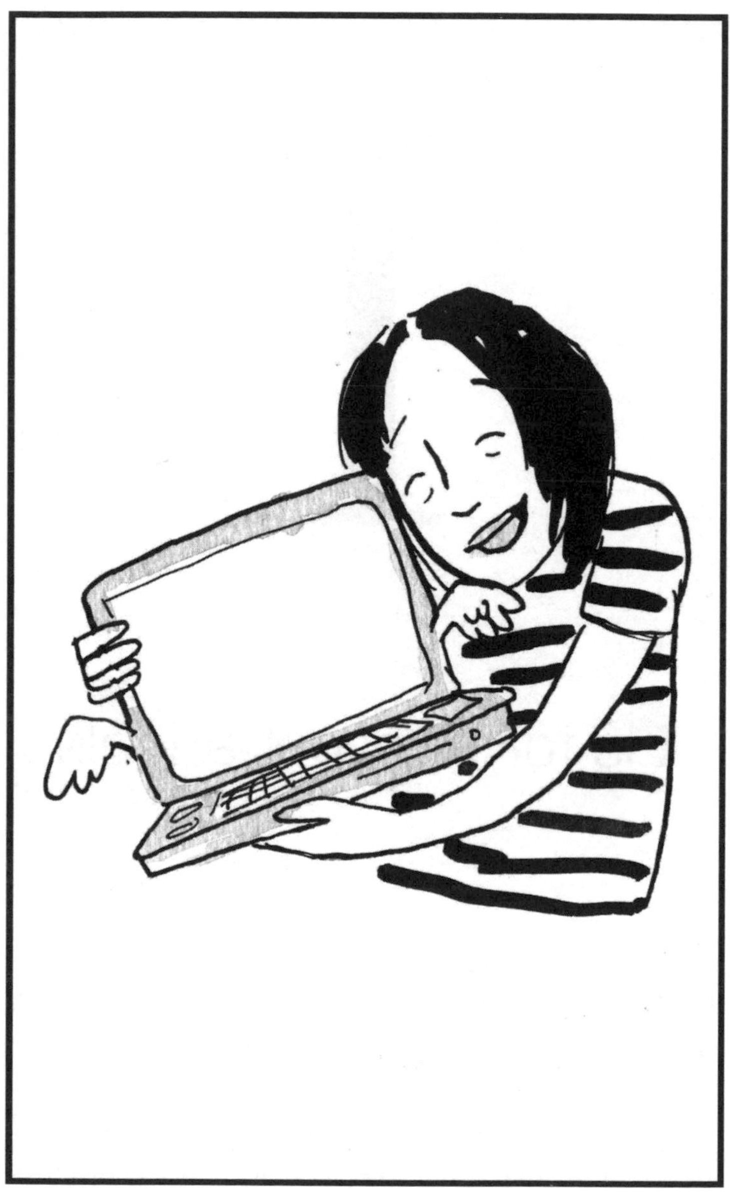

nod and we *don't* want to be told to 'relax'. But when we're TTC we need to share our stories, ask questions and talk to other women who are trying to stick it to the Baby Gods too. It's nice to sit down, offload and be there for others too. That's why the Internet is host to the biggest TTC morning tea party you'll ever be invited to. All are welcome, everyone gets a say and it's all conducted in the privacy of your own home (you don't even have to vacuum!). I call the girls in these chat rooms 'Internet angels' because you don't see them or hear them but you always know they're out there. Day or night, someone, somewhere, will be there for you.

Where to go

There are lots of great websites on fertility and pregnancy and many have forums within the site so you can chat with women in Britain or overseas. Check out a few and see what suits your own personal style before becoming a member. Some good websites to check out include:
www.britishfertilitysociety.co.uk
www.fertilityfriends.co.uk
www.babyhopes.com
www.babycentre.co.uk
www.parentsconnect.com
www.infertilitynetworkuk.com

How anonymous is it?

Chatting in TTC forums is completely anonymous until you start revealing who you are via your conversations or signatures (the photos, prose and graphics that come up every time you post). Lots of women use photographs of their pets or children in their signatures but very rarely post photos of themselves. I once read a thread where two women finally worked out they were cousins after one of them recognised a child in a photograph. They happily laughed off making the connection but I bet both secretly wondered if they should have revealed all about their husband's sperm and stories about annoying mothers-in-law so freely. There's no taking anything back online. Once it's out there, it's out there for all forum members to read.

'Whatever you do, shut down the page before your partner reads it. I once wrote a big nasty rant about him and he read it when I left the computer to make dinner. He was so pissed off!'
Sam, 33

If you want to stay completely anonymous:

- don't use any photographs at all in your signature
- use a name that sounds nothing like yours (most women go for names like Mum2B)
- don't reveal what kind of work you do or at least don't be too specific
- don't reveal where you live.

Can I get up close and personal?

Lots of women who meet online later meet up in person if they live in the same town and want the camaraderie and support in person. Just get to know your cyber friends really well before you meet up with them in person. This is the Internet – there are weirdos around, even on TTC sites.

> ‘The online community was a lifeline when I was TTC. Even though it took us over a year to conceive our second child I didn't tell a soul we were trying. I could share everything with my online friends but keep my privacy through the day in my real life.’ **Prue, 35**

Etiquette

The etiquette for posting and chatting on TTC forums is the same as for all Internet forums:

- Be polite.
- Don't be an Internet Rambo and use the space to take a swing at or dump all your anger on poor unsuspecting chatters.
- Try not to swear.
- Keep to the subject.
- Using capital letters is considered SHOUTING so only use them if you mean to shout.
- Think twice before replying when you're angry. You can't take it back once it's out there.

> 'Being online just made me see how psychotic I was getting. I stopped myself and got some actual face-to-face help with a therapist; she was wonderful.' **Lesley, 30**

Can you join several sites?

I'm a member of three, or is it four? I don't check all of them every day of course, but I pop in regularly to see what's going on. You can join as many sites as you like but perhaps stick to just one or two to really get to know fellow chatters. You'll find the same names and signatures pop up over and over and they'll soon become your friends. Some chatters are very funny while others are warm and encouraging. You'll soon find your favourites and you'll add to their TTC experience too.

> 'Just don't come back and tell everyone online to relax when you do get pregnant – they'll crucify you!' **Sam, 33**

Is it ever a nasty place?

There's a lot of emotion riding high in TTC as you know and, as with any group of women all discussing a subject they feel intimately attached to, it can lead to confrontations and some occasional bitchiness. All threads (as the separate discussion topics are known) are regulated by a moderator within the site who will disable a thread if it gets too out of control or bitchy. If someone says something you don't agree with then you don't have to correct them. If you feel angry and upset just remember to take a break from your computer before writing back. Don't post when you're angry with someone online.

It's okay to be bitchy about your real life, like when you're upset with husbands and people you work with or Smug Fertility Goddesses. In fact, other TTC-ers love it when other women vent about their real lives and how frustrating people can be – it's all part of the online therapy.

> 'Sometimes chat rooms can be a bit too hard core. They are very good for lots of women but for others they just make them worry unnecessarily. If you read anything you don't understand, ask your specialist – don't go searching online if it's just making you worry.' **IVF specialist, Dr Bill Watkins**

Is there anything you can't talk about online?

When it comes to TTC, no, there's nothing you can't talk about. You can discuss your cervical mucus, the quality of your partner's gizz and every emotional response you've ever had to the Smug Fertility Goddess in your life (is she blind?!). It's a free space and all is accepted and apologised for with a quick 'Sorry, TMI' – too much information.

However, when it comes to real life, as in your day-to-day life, then you have to be a little more careful with topics that aren't specifically about TTC. I once watched a forum thread started by a woman who suspected her husband was cheating on her. In a moment of insecurity she vented all her fears in a TTC forum. More than 780 chatters read her post and many responded telling her to leave him immediately. It all got a bit personal, bitchy and out of control as more and more opinions flooded in on what she should do or not do. Many started arguing among themselves about what was right and wrong – without even knowing the couple! No doubt it added to the poor woman's confusion and despair.

'I offend people all the time because I post when I'm tired and emotional and have my period. Thank God they don't really know me!' **Hannah, 31**

Just remember, take what you need from online forums and give back where you can too. Don't get so caught up in other people's problems that the TTC burden is even greater on your own shoulders. If it's not what you need you can always switch off the computer and walk away.

'Online women are freaky. They talk too much about their body fluids and when they have sex with their husbands. I think it's gross. But I do learn things!' **Kate, 28**

You think *your* story is complicated?

Here is a random example of one of the more complicated personal TTC stories you might find out there on the Internet – just in case you thought yours was too messy to talk about: 'My story includes a miscarriage, a mild bicornuate/ subseptate uterus, an ectopic pregnancy years ago, a dodgy tube, ovulation tracking, three IVF cycles, testing a slight positive to cardiolipin antibodies, undiagnosed but then treated endometriosis and two fertility specialists.'

Your story doesn't seem so complicated now, does it?

Do I have to say anything?

No, you can simply read the posts by others. You'll often find a post has been read, say, 400 times but only 14 people will have responded to it. And that's okay. It's like sneaking into a lecture theatre to sit up the back and listen to the teacher but not add anything to the discussion. You'll probably learn a lot about your own situation just by reading what other TTC-ers are going through and if nothing else, feel less alone.

'Sometimes the things I felt and said to my husband shocked him, like being intensely angry at someone who'd just announced they were pregnant, but they never shocked the online community.' **Donna, 36**

Does it matter how petty and bitchy I sound?

No! You can be petty, bitchy, hopeless, miserable, bitter, angry and anything else you like. It's a free space and because of the anonymity you can be whoever you like – maybe even your true self that you can't be in front of friends and family. It might be good for you!

'I went online about 20 times a day when we were TTC to talk to other women in IVF. It made me feel better that I could ask a lot of dumb questions – and I had plenty! There was always someone who knew an answer or could at least direct me where else to look.' **Kim, 37**

All the online TTC lingo you'll ever need – and then some

A

AF: Aunt Flo – your period. It's an old-school term but Aunt Flo seems to be a TTC family member online; you'll see lots of her

AI: artificial insemination

AO: anovulation

B

Babydust: good luck wishes for getting pregnant

BBs: boobs

BC: birth control

BD: baby dance (a very odd term for sex)

BF: boyfriend

BFN: big fat negative

BFP: big fat positive

C

C#: cycle number

CB: cycle buddy

CD: cycle day

CM: cervical mucus

D

DD: dear daughter (I always wonder at the 'dear' bit but there it is!)

DH: dear husband

DP: dear partner

DPO: days post-ovulation

DPT: days post-transfer

DS: dear son

Dx: diagnosis

E

EDD: estimated due date

ENDO: endometriosis

EPT: early pregnancy test

ET: embryo transfer

EW, EWCM: egg white cervical mucus

F

FET: frozen embryo transfer

FP: follicular phase

FSH: follicle stimulating hormone

G

GnRH: gonadotropin releasing hormone

GP: general practitioner

H

HPT: home pregnancy test

I

IF: infertility

IRL: in real life

IVF: in-vitro fertilisation

J

JIC: just in case

J/K: just kidding

JTYWLTK: just thought you would like to know

K

KUP: keep us posted

KWIM: know what I mean

L

LAP: laparoscopy

LH: luteinising hormone

LMP: last menstrual period (the start date)

LOL: laughing out loud

LP: luteal phase

LPD: luteal phase defect

LSP: low sperm count

M

MC, m/c: miscarriage

MF: male factor

M/S, MS: morning sickness

N

Newbie: new to Internet forums

NFP: natural family planning

O

O: ovulation, ovulated

OB: obstetrician

OB/GYN: obstetrician/ gynecologist

OPK: ovulation predictor kit

P

PCO: polycystic ovaries

PCOS: polycystic ovary syndrome

PG: pregnant

PMS: pre-menstrual syndrome

POAS: pee on a stick

(taking a home pregnancy test)

R

RE: reproductive endocrinologist

R-FSH: recombinant human follicle stimulating hormone

S

SA: semen analysis

SO: significant other

STD: sexually transmitted disease

T

TMI: too much information

TTC: trying to conceive

TWW: Two Week Wait (also 2WW)

Tx: treatment

U

UR: urologist

U/S: ultrasound

UTI: urinary tract infection

V

V: vasectomy

VR: vasectomy reversal

W

WU?: What's up?

WYSIWYG: what you see is what you get

Z

ZIFT: zygote intra-fallopian transfer

PS: Here's one I made up: LMOO (laughing my ovaries off). I hope it catches on!

Of course, you don't have to use any of these to get your message read. I didn't. My first post went something like this and maybe yours could be similar but with your own set of circumstances and questions.

> 'Hi, I'm new to this forum. We've been trying to have a baby for about a year and just had all the tests – including a laparoscopy – and everything is fine (physically). I'm getting really frustrated, over it and worried. I'm wondering if we should try to overhaul our lifestyle or jump straight into IVF as I'm 35. Any advice? Many thanks! Kind regards, Mrs Nutcase.'

No fancy acronyms needed there and I got lots of responses within an afternoon. It's not a special code, you can spell everything out if you like, just not your real name. But if you fall in love with the forums – and most who dabble do – you'll start using the TTC acronyms too in no time without really thinking about it – if you KWIM.

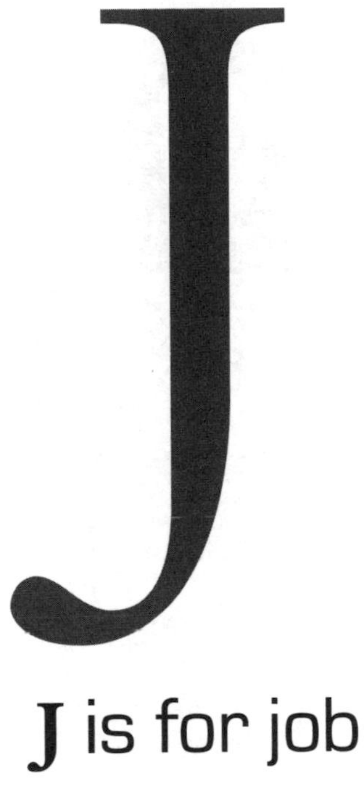

J is for job

Distracted soon-to-be mum invited to apply for exciting new position. Tasks include researching pregnancy symptoms online, loitering in the bathroom and emailing TTC friends. Applicants will need to drop the ball during the Two Week Wait and run from extra projects before going on maternity leave. If you function normally when you get your period please do not apply. Send us your CV!

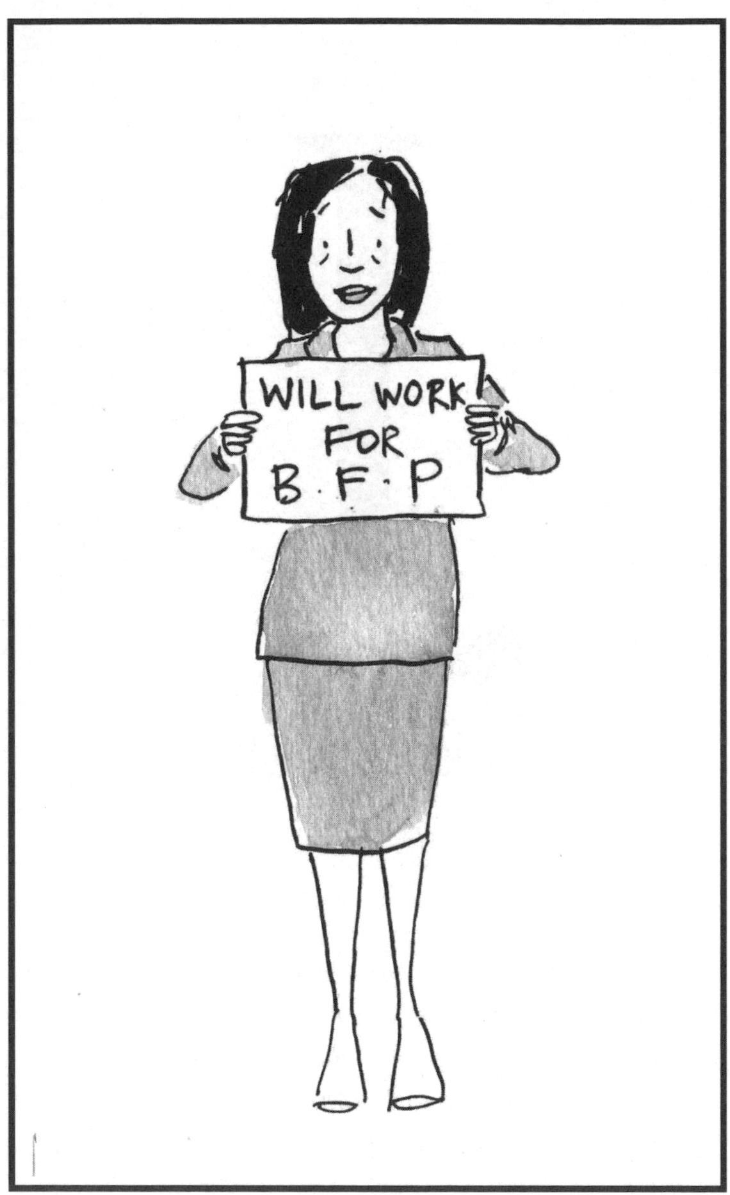
WILL WORK
FOR
B·F·P

The perfect job for me! I'm afraid I spent six months at my work with a semi-permanent scowl on my face and more time stomping off to the office bathroom than in pitch meetings (oops). Trying to get pregnant can feel like a full-time job but unfortunately most of us still have to go to work. When I finally got pregnant an unsuspecting colleague said 'You look different – you're smiling'. It was then that I realised I'd been unhappy at work for months. It's hard to be happy when you're TTC and it's taking over your relationship and your career. For me, TTC became the new career I had while still turning up to do my job. It was hard work.

'I started a new job right after we started trying for a baby. I knew it was the right time to have a baby and I just couldn't worry too much about letting people down or being distracted at work. You just have to follow your heart and hope the rest turns out okay.' **Kate, 28**

Getting organised at work

Being organised during office hours will help you get through your working week and you can even plan to have TTC time at work – without falling behind.

First of all, email. Can you resist responding to every email that flies in every five minutes? Perhaps make a time in the day (say, when you first arrive at 9 a.m.) to respond to emails and then leave your inbox alone until the end of the day – unless of course email is directly a part of your work. Don't spend the day emailing colleagues across the room or hanging out in the kitchen wasting time. Make a meeting time, cover everything you need to for the day and perhaps tell them you're not checking email as religiously as you used to. Hold off on emailing friends back until the next morning and don't bother about sending on email chains or opening joke emails. Delete, delete, delete.

Streamline your desk inbox too. Clear out what is no longer needed and work out what has to be done and when. Prioritise your workload. Schedule in faux 'meetings' or let someone know you won't be at your desk so you can use an OPK (ovulation predictor kit) at 2 p.m. in the office bathroom.

Limit your perusing of TTC sites to no more than an hour of your day! That doesn't mean two minutes checking here, 10 minutes there. Give yourself a solid hour to catch up on posts and post some of your own. And then leave it. Go back to work!

Networking, what's that again?

There was a time when work was exciting and turning up to networking functions with wine, cheese on sticks and stale crackers was great fun. When you're TTC, a lot of women will tell you that the chit-chat has dried up, their small talk skills have evaporated and they just don't care anymore. I stopped going to every work function outside work hours when we were TTC because I just couldn't be bothered. I felt as if I should've worn a badge with 'Sorry, distracted' or 'Desperately want to go on maternity leave' the entire year before I actually *did* go on maternity leave. However, if networking and mixing and mingling are part of your job then you might just have to turn up to a few events. If you have to go, create an excuse to leave early; have one drink, speak to everyone you're supposed to and then sneak out of there.

The TTC sickie

I am all for 'pulling a sickie' when you just can't face the world and only the ladies on *Loose Women* cut it for company. Not every week but every now and then it's nice to call in sick to work and just spend the day alone, on the couch or in the garden and not in the grind of work. As soon as you've made the call, forgive yourself immediately for being a no-show and forget about what needs to be done at the office (otherwise you may as well go in!). The TTC sickie is just another little way of keeping yourself calm and happy through the month. If you just can't seem to find the time to unwind but you know in your heart (and BlackBerry) that you must slow down here and there in order to get pregnant, just *take* the time.

> 'Working with pregnant women is torture when you're TTC. Ours is a big office with lots of women and I can't escape them. I act really busy and pretend to be on the phone so I won't have to chat about baby things.' **Holly, 34**

TTC handbag stuffers

Part of being organised is ensuring you have the following TTC items with you at work:

- ovulation predictor kit
- bag of zinc-packed sunflower and pumpkin seeds to munch on
- supplements you might need to take at lunchtime
- fertility-friendly herbal tea bags such as peppermint, lemon, and lemongrass and ginger
- list of emergency stress-busters (see 'Stress busting at work' on page 132) – in case you forget!
- the Bump & Grind Diary (see 'K is for keeping track' for one of those).

Staying emotionally unavailable

Funny how TTC can become the career that you now can't believe you used to go on about. But careers take a whole lot of emotional input to push them forward. They take commitment, desire and punctuality – even when you get your period. If the passion you once felt for your career has well and truly left the building for now, that's okay. But instead of feeling guilty and *half* keeping up with it all emotionally (which is exhausting), give yourself a break and allow yourself to be emotionally unavailable. It's okay not to be 100 per cent into your job – so long as you're not letting the team down or risking losing your income. But if you feel that familiar banging and clanging of alarm bells that you should be doing more, more, more and it's making you feel stressed, stop yourself, take a moment to breathe and stretch.

> 'Giving up my obsession with work was the best thing I did in TTC! It was too hard being a good colleague knowing I was desperate to be on maternity leave. I didn't let anyone know but inside I let myself stop caring about work.' **Kim, 37**

Dealing with dickheads at work

You know who they are. There's the guy who warns you you'd better 'Squeeze out a few puppies' because you're not getting any younger. The older woman who tells you she feels desperately sorry for 30-something career women without children – as babies are 'the greatest gift of all from the universe' (ugh).

There are also the dickheads who you know in your heart aren't really dickheads but they put their foot in it anyway. When a male colleague of mine asked me a few years ago if Ben and I were trying to have a baby, I waved him away with a vague 'maybe' and he went on to tell me how easy it was for him to knock up his wife back in the day, to which I accidentally snapped 'Good for you!' The next day he came over to see if he'd 'hit a bum note' with me, then said 'For all I know you're secretly having an awful time getting pregnant, just like a family friend of ours who tried for five years. It ruined her marriage and her life, really, they ended up divorced – anyway, best of luck!' I. Was. Floored. Try to stay away from people and conversations where TTC might come up. Change the topic. Ask *them* a horridly personal question and see how they run.

Do you tell your boss you're TTC?

That of course depends on your boss and his or her need to know. If you're going through IVF and having to leave work for scans during work hours then it might be worth confiding in your boss that that's where you are sneaking off to. There are two risks here: one, that your fertility troubles will end up office gossip; and two, you'll be sent to Mummyville and not considered for future promotions because your boss knows you are trying to have a baby and will eventually apply for maternity leave. A fair, understanding and generous boss would be a godsend when you're TTC but they are a rarity. Unless of course *you're* the boss – then give yourself permission to fall behind!

> 'I told my boss I was TTC when she found me crying in the bathroom (I got my period). From that day on she treated me with special attention and let me take an afternoon off here and there. She'd gone through IVF five years earlier.'
>
> **Heather, 36**

The office bathroom

The times I have cried in the office bathroom! Like the time I started bleeding mid-cycle. And the time I found out a former colleague was pregnant (again!). Or the time I couldn't focus on a story I was writing because the Two Week Wait was driving me crazy and I missed the deadline.

Crying in the office bathroom is perfectly acceptable when you're TTC. If you feel a flood of tears coming on just make sure you reach the safety of a bathroom cubicle before they spill over or you might be followed by a sweet colleague you probably don't want to confide in. Paper soaked in cold water will help with red puffy eyes. And don't venture out until you're ready. I once spent 30 minutes crying in the bathroom – you can imagine how I looked at the end of it: hello panda eyes!

‘I sometimes Google information on getting pregnant, print it out, sneak it under my jacket and go and read it in the privacy of the bathroom cubicle. I don’t want anyone seeing what I’m reading or asking dumb questions at work.’

Sam, 33

Ovulation testing at work

The best time to use an OPK (ovulation predictor kit) is 2 p.m. Don’t drink too much water in the hour before you test – it’ll dilute your urine. Give yourself plenty of time in the bathroom cubicle. Don’t chat with someone washing their hands, they may wait for you to finish.

Be stealthy. The test will take about seven minutes to complete. It might be one of those situations where you have to take your handbag into the bathroom with you, so perhaps pretend to be leaving the building and duck into the bathroom on your way. Now that’s stealthy.

‘Every time I got my period when I was at work I would get out of the office at lunchtime and buy shoes. I have an awesome collection of boots. I call them my Screw You Boots.’ **Karen, 38**

TTC-friendly lunchtime ideas

- Join the gym and go to a fun class or just use the treadmill.
- Go to a yoga class.
- Sit in a park or a grassy spot to eat your lunch.
- Have a fertility-friendly ginger tea with a friend.
- Buy baby clothes if it cheers you up and motivates you – but not if it bums you out!
- Try not to stare sadly at young mums and pregnant women on the street (they're probably thinking how good *you* have it!).
- Visit your favourite homewares shop and salivate over all the tasty appliances.
- Go shopping for your husband and surprise him (*Karma Sutra* perhaps?).

'I *love* shopping for baby clothes during my lunch hour. It cheers me up. I don't buy anything too expensive. Besides, I'm going to need it all soon!' **Kate, 28**

Am I stressed or just busy?

Getting everything done on time is different to getting everything splattered on when your head explodes. Some symptoms of work-related stress include depression, anxiety, feeling overwhelmed, sleeping problems, an increase in (genuine) sick days, fatigue and headaches. If that sounds like you then it's definitely time to slow down your work pace and get some balance back. If you're feeling overly rushed and frazzled then it's time to stop and see what's really important. Scale back, take a break, learn to say no to colleagues, friends and family who may all want a piece of you.

> 'I sometimes think that if I could go and live on a tropical island for three months then maybe I'd get pregnant. The daily stresses of work are really hard on my body and my emotions. I sometimes wonder if that's all it is preventing a pregnancy – work stress.' **Holly, 34**

Stress busting at work

- Get organised (come in on a weekend to – finally! – clean up your desk).
- Don't let things pile up.
- Don't get involved in office gossip and time-wasting drama.
- Don't get too far behind – ask for help.
- Be mindful of the lighting – you don't want any glare on your computer screen or to be sitting under a flickering fluorescent light.
- Get out of the office at lunchtime and go for a walk.
- Eat healthy lunches and snacks and drink lots of water throughout the day (have a 2-litre bottle of water on your desk to remind yourself to drink it).

- Don't have more than one coffee a day max.
- Give yourself regular breaks – stand up and walk around.
- Go grab some fresh air.
- Don't ignore the signs of stress.

PS: If you're struggling at work, remember: maternity leave is just around the corner – you'll be the boss of the pantry and the couch! Oh, and the baby.

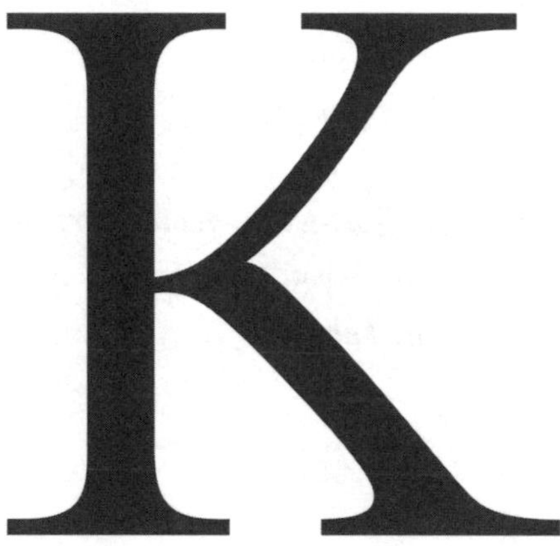

K is for keeping track

That little egg of yours is a party girl. She'll be on a 24-hour mission to get hit on by your husband's best player and then she'll be gone. You can't know exactly what night she'll be loitering in your fallopian tube so you might want to keep track of your cycle throughout the month. Keeping track can also help you feel in control.

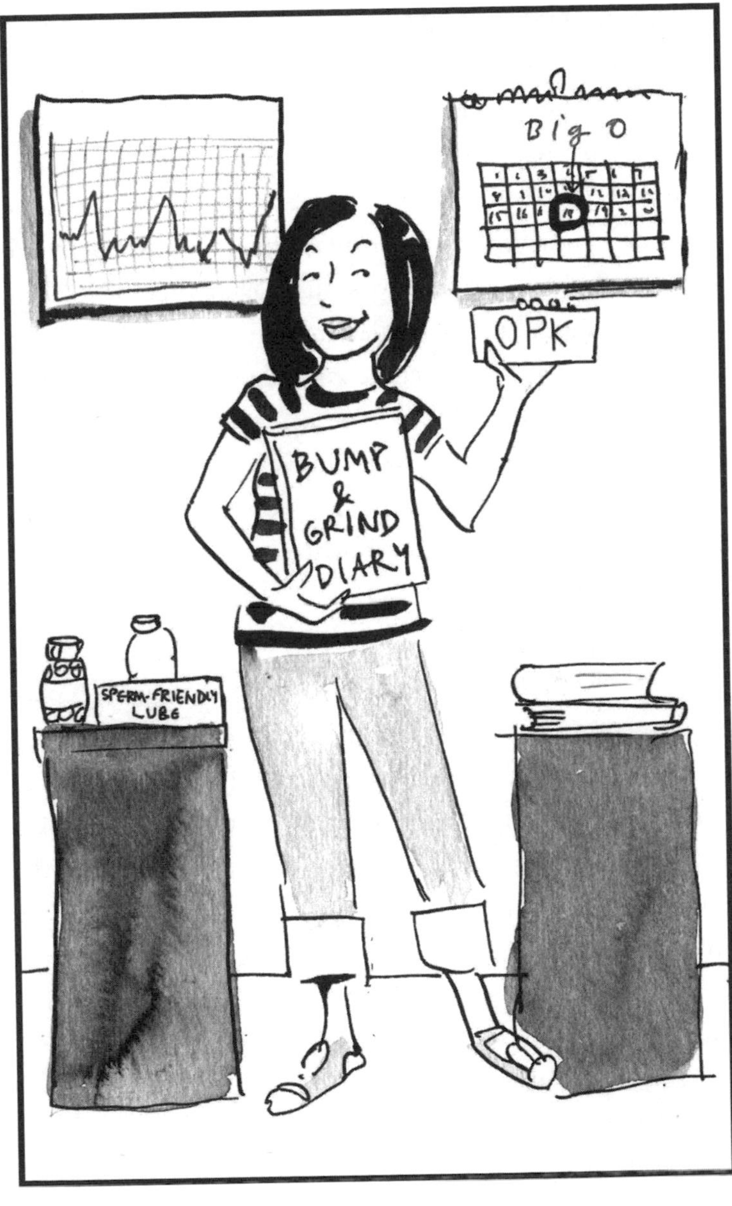
Big O
OPK
BUMP & GRIND DIARY
SPERM-FRIENDLY LUBE

Locating 'the window'

The Fertile Window provides the best possible view to conceiving. It's generally considered to be the three days before ovulation, ovulation day itself and then three days afterwards. You want plenty of bump and grind in that seven-day timeframe. And you can pick and choose how you'd like to monitor your cycle and work out when ovulation is likely to occur. You can use an ovulation predictor kit and let your urine tell you; you can chart your temperature for a few months and let that tell you; you can keep a very close eye on your cervical mucus; or you can wait 'til you're horny and let *that* be your guide … Of course, you can use all of these. That party girl doesn't stand a chance!

The Bump & Grind Diary

A TTC friend tells me that keeping track of her cycle gave her something to do which helped pass the time and keep her sane through the first two weeks of the month (she was a *bit* bonkers during the Two Week Wait – aren't we all?). You can create a lot of TTC busy work – complete with the Bump & Grind Diary, a few new pens, a new highlighter, gold stickers and maybe some glitter glue … Buy yourself a special new journal or notebook. TTC is a challenging but exciting time – it's worth having a beautiful new diary for.

To get you started, record the following:

- the date
- cycle day

- morning temperature on your basal body temperature (BBT) chart
- state of cervical mucus
- cervix position (hard or soft – see page 142)
- OPK result (if using)
- list of fertility super foods you've eaten today
- record of any exercise you've done today
- your weight
- feelings/emotions (including any angry, bitter, nasty, defeated, bitchy, negative thoughts – better out than in!)
- positive thoughts/affirmations
- sex report (as in, did you do it?)

And that's just one day!

> 'Keeping a record of everything was my way of being in control of a situation that felt out of control. I loved my TTC diary, I took it everywhere and wrote daily updates. It was a good way to keep track of my emotional stuff too.' **Sam, 33**

The Big O

Remember when the Big O was about orgasm? When you're TTC it's about ovulation which is a tad more boring but vital to know about when getting pregnant. Now, if you're like me, most of what we learnt in school biology class about menstruation and ovulation got lost somewhere between a goth teen phase and the grunge twenties phase when it was all about *not* getting pregnant. Who cared about ovulation? It was just something that probably happened every month no matter how flat your chest was so long as you were getting periods. So when we start out TTC most of us need a crash course in ovulation.

Back to biology

Ovulation is when an egg (occasionally more than one) is released from the ovary. Each month an egg matures inside your ovary and once it reaches a certain size it gets swept into the fallopian tube towards the uterus. The egg lives for 24 hours (enough time to put on her shoes and her favourite lippie and to get out there and see which sperm hits on her first). Ovulation occurs only once a month. The time in the month at which it occurs can vary but it generally happens 14 days before the end of your cycle. If you have a 28-day cycle then ovulation is probably on or around day 14. But it can vary from month to month and take longer to release the egg (she can't decide which shoes to wear), depending sometimes on what's going on in your daily life. In her book *Taking Charge of Your Fertility*, Toni Weschler says you should never rely on day 14 as a guide to ovulation. 'In actuality,' writes Weschler, 'ovulation *may* occur on day 14; it may also occur on day 10, day 18, or day 37. In other words, ovulation is not the consistent event it is presumed to be.' But there are tools and techniques to know exactly when your party girl egg will be out and about and when to send in the sperm for a dance. Here's a general overview.

Ovulation predictor kits (OPKs)

Ovulation predictor kits or OPKs detect the surge in luteinising hormone (LH) in your urine just before ovulation. They can predict ovulation 12 to 36 hours in advance. So if you have a 28-day cycle you'd start testing from day 11. If your cycle runs between 27 and 34 days your ovulation range might be day 13 to day 20. So start testing on day 11 and keep testing until day 20.

The best time to test is at 2 p.m. or as close as possible. Anytime between noon and 8 p.m. is still fine. First morning urine is not recommended because it can take up to four hours for LH to show up in your urine. Most women will ovulate 12 to 48 hours after the LH surge is detected – the most common is 36 hours after the actual surge. Don't drink lots of water in the few hours before you test – you don't want to dilute your urine.

You can buy OPKs at the chemist for about £20 for a box of seven but when you're hardcore TTC you might want to buy them online – without the fancy packaging and just as good – a whole lot cheaper.

OPK sample sex schedule

What do you do when you get a positive OPK result? You have sex! And then you do it again the next day. Here's a sex schedule as put together by my TTC friend Cath, 34, who got pregnant on the second cycle using an OPK.

1. Have sex as soon as you see that line and the LH surge is detected. Even though you will probably ovulate 12 to 36 hours later, you want the sperm 'up there' when the egg comes down.
2. Have sex twice on the day *after* you see the surge (once first thing in the morning and then about eight hours later).
3. Have 'insurance sex' the next morning and the one after that too.

'I wasn't having any luck until I got an OPK at the chemist and some PreSeed online and said to my partner 'Okay, this is it!' The idea is to get the sperm up there before the egg comes down and then flood the area with fresh sperm on the following days. You want the sperm cruising inside good mucus so if you don't think you have the right sort, get PreSeed. You can't know exactly what time the egg will be there so you have to give yourself lots and lots of chances. This worked for us – on the second cycle. It also worked for a friend of mine who had been trying for over a year. I was going to say good luck – but you won't need it!! Try it out this month.' **Cath, 34**

PS: Don't forget, sperm often has the most 'mojo' in the morning.

Basal body temperature (BBT)

Your temperature fluctuates throughout the month in accordance with where you are in your cycle. So while charting your temperature alone won't tell you when to have sex this month, over a few months you'll be able to tell on which day you normally ovulate.

Just before ovulation your temperature will dip slightly. You are most likely to ovulate on the day you see your temperature take a dip. The temperature should then spike the next day, indicating ovulation has occurred. For example, if you get a temperature hike on day 15 of your cycle you can predict you ovulated on day 14. For the first half of your cycle (the follicular phase) your temperature should be low – usually between 36.1°C and 36.6°C. After ovulation you enter the second half of the cycle (the luteal phase) where your temperature can range from 36.7°C to 37°C. It will begin to drop again before the start of your period. If you are pregnant your temperature will stay high and can range from 36.9°C to 37.3°C.

To chart all this action you need a basic digital thermometer that measures temperature in tenth degrees – like 37.2. Take your temperature before you get out of bed every morning. It's best to take your temperature after at least four straight hours of sleep. Any illness, insomnia or alcohol consumption the night before can affect your temperature.

Saliva ovulation microscope

This little contraption looks like fun. It's a microscope the size of a lipstick that fits neatly in your purse. It's a saliva test you do every day to see when your oestrogen rises and ovulation is imminent. Here's how it works. The level of oestrogen in saliva rises dramatically in the two to three days before ovulation. Through the microscope an 'oestrogen phase' looks like ferns. In a 'transitional' phase you will see pebbles. I have TTC friends who swear by this tricky device although I quite often got a construction site scene that was hard to distinguish ... You can buy a saliva ovulation test kit online for about £20. You use it every day before you eat or drink anything (water is fine). The trick is to get enough saliva on the lens to get a result but nothing so gob-like that it doesn't dry in 10 minutes. Anything over ten minutes is an invalid reading.

Cervical position

The position of the cervix changes throughout your cycle. That's why sex sometimes feels easy and comfortable (you're probably in the Fertile Window) and not so comfortable a few weeks later (an infertile time). How do you know? You can feel it.

Before you dive in: wash your hands; cut any long nails; sit on the toilet or stand with one foot on the bath; take a deep breath. Does your cervix feel low or high in your vagina? At the start of your cycle your cervix should feel low and hard (it'll feel like the tip of your nose). As ovulation gets closer your cervix will begin to rise and soften (it'll feel more like your lips).

PS: If you want your partner to assess the position of your cervix I've read the best position is by leaning down 'on your hands and knees while your partner checks you from behind'. Hmm, there's close in TTC and then there's too close.

Cervical mucus

It is with a few giggles that we get to the vital topic of cervical mucus, a term so icky and unsexy that in her book *Taking Charge of Your Fertility,* Toni Weschler renames it 'cervical fluid'. Let's stick with mucus just for laughs. Okay, so the *mucus* changes throughout your cycle, letting you know when you are fertile and when you are at a non-fertile time in your cycle. It generally goes like this:

Mucus before ovulation

The first few days after your period there will be little or no discharge. You will feel dryness around your vulva (your what-now?! Your vulva!). The chances of getting pregnant at this time are low.

PS: The vulva is the whole external genitalia of your body including the labia majora and minora. Hmm, I wasn't sure about that either ...

Mucus approaching ovulation

Discharge is moist and sticky and is most probably white or cream in colour. It should break up easily in your fingers. In this transition time the mucus will get slightly cloudy, stretch more easily and there'll be more of it.

Mucus right around the Big O

You hear a lot about egg whites in TTC and this is what they are talking about. The mucus now should look like egg white and stretch between your fingers. There is reportedly a 'mucus peak' somewhere around this time but really, who has time to wait around for that? The sperm loves egg white mucus and can survive in this magical goop for up to 72 hours. If your egg is out and about waiting for The One special sperm to hit on her then there's an excellent chance pregnancy will occur.

Mucus after ovulation

After such dizzy heights, the mucus goes back to being sticky, and again there is a feeling of dryness around the vulva.

Much-loved mucus boosters

Try taking any of these to help thin out the mucus, create more mucus – or both!:

- green tea
- grapeseed extract
- salty foods such as popcorn (mucus contains a lot of salt)
- *lots* of water.

It's also a good idea to speak to your naturopath who may have other suggestions to boost your mucus-making.

But *how* do I check the cervical mucus?

With your fingers. Some women get really handy at poking about their cervix to check on their cervical mucus. Cut your fingernails first! Do not, I repeat, do not ask your partner how things 'feel' mucus-wise down there. He may just lose his lunch and most definitely his erection.

Ovulation pain

Ovulation pain is often referred to as 'mittelschmerz' which sounds like something you might say after too many drinks. Alas, it's a German word for 'middle pain' and affects many women every cycle or more commonly every third or fourth cycle.

What can it feel like?

A sharp twinge diminishing into a dull ache (usually in your right side); cramping; nausea; increased urination. Ovulation pain can last for six to eight hours in most women or even up to 24 to 48 hours. It's caused by a small leakage of blood from the ovary at ovulation time which can cause an irritation of the abdominal wall.

> 'I'd never really noticed ovulation pain but when I was paying attention to it – the pain in one side, feeling slightly sick – it seemed so obvious. Now I know my exact dates.' **Kate, 28**

PS: I once asked a TTC friend exactly how she knew when she was ovulating when she didn't use an OPK and she said 'Puh-lease, I was horny!'

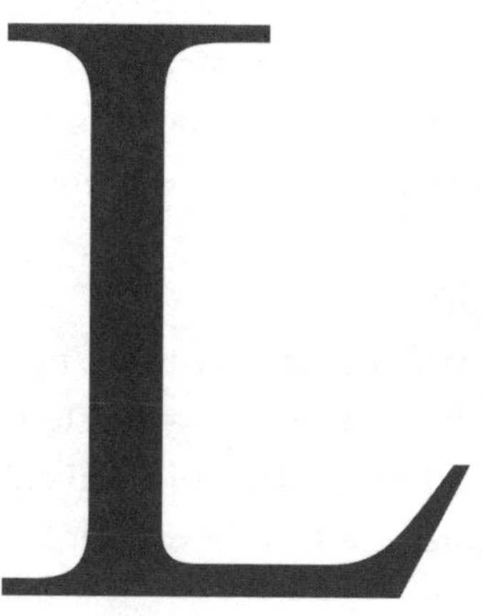

L is for last time and getting 'lapped'

Anyone who has battled the Baby Gods knows that wanting a baby is *wanting a baby* no matter how old you are, if you already have children or if you have just started popping the folic acid and hanging upside down. *Wanting a baby is wanting a baby.* Therefore it's upsetting and unfair that secondary

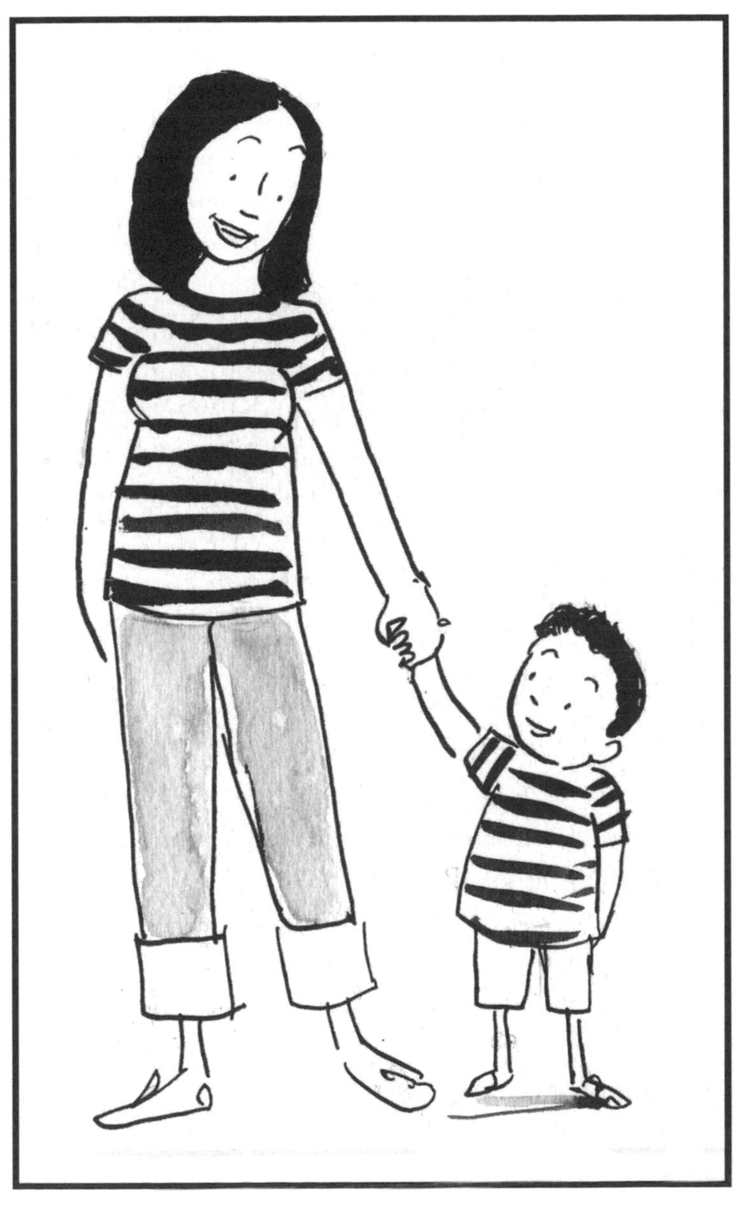

infertility (when a couple struggles to have a second child) isn't generally considered as traumatic as primary infertility.

Secondary infertility reportedly accounts for as many as 60 per cent of infertility cases. Most people assume if you have already proved yourself in the fertility stakes the first time around then you'll be able to do it again. But it isn't always the case. Many couples don't go for fertility treatment because they just don't assume anything could be wrong. Most couples are also told by well-meaning relatives and even doctors to stop worrying and just keep trying. But when you're not only battling the Baby Gods but biology too (tick tock, tick tock – grr!) it might be smart to have some basic tests done too.

So what may have changed since last time you got pregnant?

- You're a little older.
- You or your partner may have had an infection or a sexually transmitted disease.
- You may have gained weight.
- You may be eating more unhealthy foods.
- You may be more stressed.
- You may have a different partner (new sperm, new ball game, so to speak).
- You may be drinking more alcohol or coffee.

Last time

Lots of women find it easy to conceive their first child but 'hit a wall' the second time around. The waiting and wanting can be unbearable. Especially when these women are already committed to mummy events like dropping toddlers at childcare or taking them to parties where everyone wants to know 'Are you having another?'

> 'I felt extreme guilt that I was so preoccupied with trying for baby number two I was missing out on focusing on the one child that I did have. I felt even more guilt that I had already been so lucky to have one at all, yet I was basically saying to myself 'he isn't enough'.' **Prue, 35**

A TTC friend of mine says secondary infertility was more painful than trying to conceive her first child because she so desperately wanted to give her child a sibling to play with and didn't want the age gap to be too great. Some say they're just 'not done' with baby-making yet. They want more.

> 'I found that I couldn't escape it as I was already immersed in that world. All the mums with children around the same age as my son were all starting to fall pregnant with their next baby. I found it all suffocating.' **Prue, 35**

If conceiving your first child was a walk in the park, sorry, a romp in the hay, then taking a long time to conceive the second can be confusing and frustrating. It might be harder to admit that you might need help because you didn't have any problems before. Lots of couples think they just need to give it more time, only the longer it takes, the more they worry which adds to the stress of TTC. Meanwhile, their child is getting older and the gap between future siblings is greater. So what could it be?

Possible causes for infertility

The following figures are from the British Human Fertilisation and Embryology Authority:

- low sperm count (32 per cent)
- tubal damage in woman (16.6 per cent)
- an ovulatory problem (4.9 per cent)
- endometriosis or another condition affecting the uterus (3.3 per cent)
- a combination of factors in both partners (17 per cent).

In 20 per cent of cases the cause of infertility (both primary and secondary infertility) is not identified, which as we've already seen is called 'unexplained infertility'. However, according to www.babycentre.co.uk, up to two-thirds of couples with unexplained infertility conceive within three years if they continue trying.

> 'Friends and acquaintances announcing more pregnancies made me feel like other women were taking my turn in the queue, as if every woman who got pregnant again was making it longer and longer until it would happen for me.' **Prue, 35**

Going for some simple fertility tests might be a smart move and don't worry if you feel like you're jumping the gun. If you want answers now – get them (see 'G is for getting on with tests and treatment'). It doesn't mean you need help this time or that you're committing to treatment. It just means you'll get some answers so you can keep up working on baby number two with a clearer mind.

Meanwhile, get off my back!

As soon as you're married, people want to know when you're having a baby and, as soon as your baby is a year old, people want to know when you're having another one. Why do people ask us to rush through our lives? Regardless, it's annoying when you are having a hard time conceiving number two and people assume when you have one that you will automatically pop out another in 15 months' time.

Plus, just like the 'us and them' mentality between those who do have a baby and those who do not, there's often an assumption that women TTC for their second should feel *grateful* they already have a child. That they should just be happy with their lot and stop complaining. And that's not fair.

> 'Just because you have been blessed with a child doesn't make the frustration in trying to conceive again any less valid.' **Sam, 33**

White lies when you're trying for number two

'We're so busy taming this toddler – another one?'
'We're giving it a year or two – there's no rush.'
'We haven't really thought about it yet.'
'We'll let you know if we ever have news to share.'
'Are you crazy? It nearly killed me the first time I gave birth!'
'Maybe in a year or two.'
'I recently read that "one is the new two"'.

Getting lapped

This is when couples you know are having their *second* baby when you are still trying for your first. It is particularly painful when those closest to you – like best friends, sisters and sisters-in-law – are having such success and you're still not there (yet!). It can be a confronting time and it's hard not to panic. I got lapped quite a few times and each time

I discovered a friend or a friend of a friend was having another baby I wanted to run and hide from the world. It just wasn't fair!

But getting lapped also made the experience of *finally* getting pregnant even more triumphant (not smug!) than it may have been without our fertility issues. When it was finally my turn I enjoyed every second of it. And you will too. Much more than the Smug Fertility Goddesses we know who – oops – accidentally got pregnant after washing their husband's Speedos. It was like I had worked so hard for it I deserved to enjoy it completely. Even when I was so tired in the first trimester I couldn't get off the couch or when my boobs drooped so suddenly in the third trimester I was practically tucking them into my super-high maternity pants, I still loved every second of it. I felt like I had *deserved* my dream. And you will too (maybe without the high pants).

Meanwhile, you really don't have to go to every baby shower or toddler's birthday party if it's too upsetting. You can be angry and sad and kick things around (maybe not your husband) but make sure you spend lots of time striving to be happy with things – just the way they are.

M

M is for more sex!

Nooooo! Not more sex! Somewhere between the Best Unprotected Sex Ever and Oh God, Not You Again, TTC throws a spanner in your sex life (and then the whole toolbox). Sex can feel routine, precise, and so well timed and executed you could take on the Russians at gymnastics (and they're not sexy). However, one of the biggest mistakes most

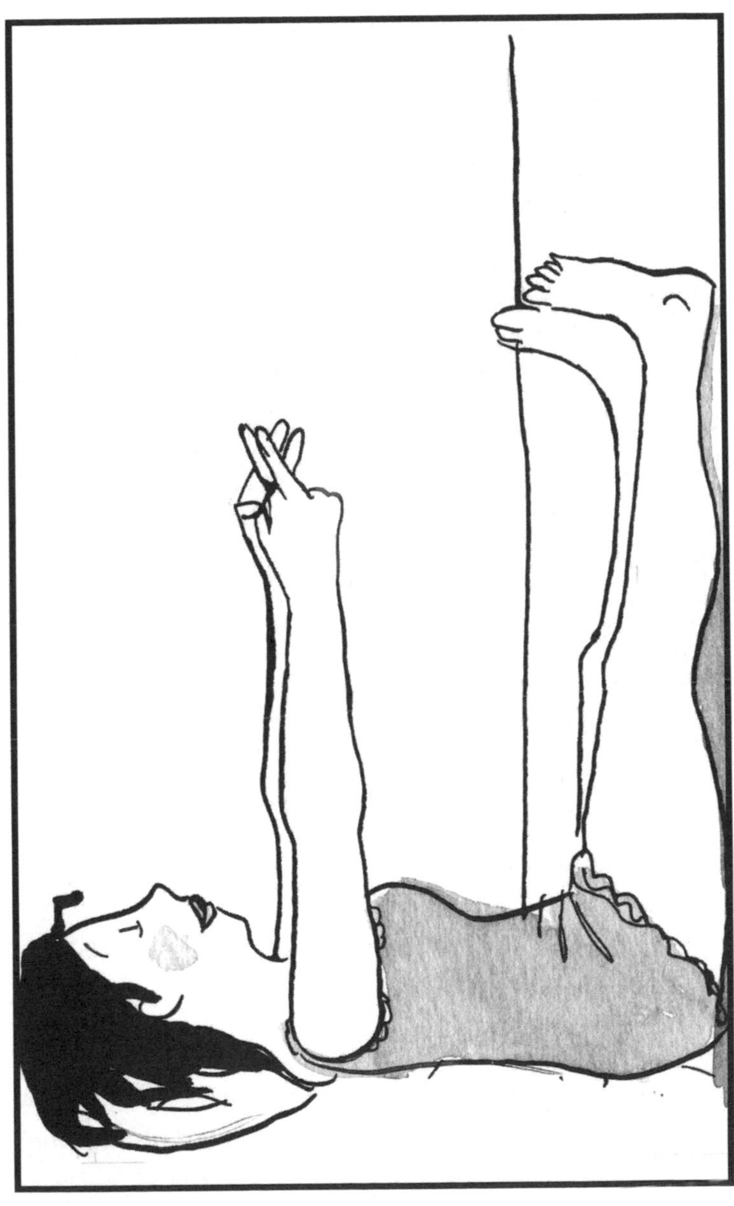

of us make when TTC is not having *enough* sex during the Fertile Window.

You have to do it often, all the time, a lot, okay, *like bunny rabbits.* I can hear you groaning – and not with ecstasy. It's not so easy when the last thing you feel like is being *easy.* It can be hard work! Plus, we girls don't help the situation. A TTC friend tells me she once whispered to her husband during sex, 'Aim for the back wall honey.' Ick! The back wall? I think she was talking about her cervix. Anyone who has been TTC for more than five months knows that baby-making sex is just different to regular sex. Regular recreational sex is all about the beginning – the foreplay, the kissing and the groping bit. When you are TTC, it's all about the Big Finish (ejaculation) and legs up ladies!

Quick Quiz: Is the romance dead?

1. Romance, you ask – who cares?
2. Have you started doing it on the couch because *Mad Men* is on TV and you don't want to leave the living room?
3. Does making out feel decadent?
4. Is reaching for the sperm-friendly lubricant considered foreplay?

If you answered 'yes' to most of the above then yep, the romance should be stuffed and placed on your mantle. If you answered 'no' to most of the above then you probably won't be found in your socks making love during the ad breaks.

> 'Instead of stressing, try to enjoy the bonking and chill out.' **Karen, 38**

Ready, set, sex!

If you want to take the pressure off tedious TTC sex try this:

- Forget about doing it exclusively in bed.
- You don't need to start or stay in the missionary position, just end up there.
- Make each other laugh.
- Forgive each other for 'boring' sex – all sex counts in TTC.
- Don't get too uptight that it has to be *exactly* 6 p.m. – or 4 a.m.
- Don't get uptight if the romance is dead.
- Don't nag him verbally for sex – go straight for his pants.

And if you're feeling daring and want to spice things up, try these:

- Plan a weekend shag-fest away from home where there is nothing on the agenda but sex.
- Try some erotic massage.
- Role play (you know, he can be the fireman, you be the nurse – mmm firemen!).
- Use kinky toys – if that's your bag.

Sexy food

If you're daring, feeding each other sexy aphrodisiacs could be a tasty way to spice things up. Aphrodisiac foods include figs, oysters, pomegranates and, would you believe, garlic. Hmm, I'm not sure a spoonful of minced garlic is too sexy. Maybe stick to the figs and pomegranates served with ice cream and follow up with bubbly (just one glass!).

Location, location

The idea is to get the sperm as close to the cervix at ejaculation as possible. Remember my friend who said, 'Aim for the back wall, honey' during sex? Well, she had a point. Good old missionary will deposit the sperm closest to the cervix. Doing it doggy-style is also an option. Forget about you on top (think gravity!). But no, don't bother doing it standing on your head or in any way upside down. That's just silly.

Legs on the wall

Riding an imaginary bike, scissor kicking the ceiling or practising water ballet straight after sex – most TTC-ers have their own moves to 'trap' the sperm and give it a good head start on getting into your uterus and hitting on your egg. But does it work? How much help does sperm need? Staying horizontal for at least 20 minutes afterwards will reportedly keep the sperm in your hoo-ha longer, but keep in mind there are millions of them in every ejaculation.

So no sleeping with your legs on the wall? It's up to you. If swinging your legs up after sex makes you feel like you're doing everything you can to help get pregnant, then do it. Some women swear by a gentle 'bike ride' with their legs in the air after sex.

Let me tell you the secrets of a friend of mine who has three children who were all conceived exactly like this: Straight after he ejaculates (in the missionary position) keep him inside you for as long as possible like a plug (how romantic!). Afterwards, gently place a folded pillow under your butt and go peacefully off to sleep trying not to move your butt around too much. Not as much fun as scissor kicking the ceiling but it did work for her – three times! Healthy, fired up sperm doesn't need that much help getting to the right spot but tilting your butt up for at least 20 minutes will help.

'I have to say I don't get any pleasure from massive amounts of sex all at once. I'd rather just try to do it twice around ovulation and cross my fingers – and my legs.' **Hannah, 31**

Gourmet sex

According to an article in *The Observer*, there is such a thing as 'gourmet sex' that will make a pregnancy more likely than tedious TTC sex. It's all about enhancing the man's pleasure in order to boost sperm count. According to the article, men produce about 250 million sperm during intercourse but those enjoying 'gourmet sex' will boost that by up to 50 per cent. Three hundred and seventy-five million sperm!

'Couples who are trying to have a baby often mention that the sex becomes a bit of a chore, a bit mechanical and routine. That's the wrong thing to be doing,' says Dr Allan Pacey, secretary of the British Fertility Society and senior lecturer in andrology at Sheffield University. 'The sex should be as wild and thrilling as it was when they first met, when they weren't thinking about babies, to give them the maximum possible chance of having a baby.'

In the same article, American expert in reproductive physiology Dr Joanna Ellington agrees: 'The better the sex, the better the chances of conception.' 'One of the things that men don't realise is that the more excited they are, the further back in the testicle they are going to draw on reserves of sperm,' she says. 'So if you have gourmet sex, where you really spend time and make it fun for both partners, that is going to make the man more stimulated and he is going to ejaculate more and healthier sperm.'

> 'Since we've been trying my partner seems so much sexier, he has a different kind of appeal now that I didn't see before we were TTC. It just really feels like we're in this together – which makes our sex better. Plus, we do it so often we really know what the other one likes!' **Sam, 33**

Should I have an orgasm?

Yes, yes, yes it is possible that uterine contractions help move sperm along the fallopian tubes after an orgasm. But such contractions reportedly happen involuntarily around ovulation anyway. Dr Pacey (of the gourmet sex article) says the female orgasm definitely enhances your chances. 'When a woman experiences an orgasm, we think the intensity of the muscular contractions she has during the big pressure changes going on in her body helps to pull or suck up the sperm into her cervix and from there into the uterus,' he says. In his book *Getting Pregnant: A compassionate resource to overcoming infertility,* Professor Robert Jansen says: 'Female orgasm *before* ejaculation decreases sperm retention, whereas orgasm *after* ejaculation can reduce flow back and increase sperm retention'. In his book *Fit For Fertility*, Dr Michael Dooley says 'Traditional Chinese medicine teaches that simultaneous orgasm will pull more of the man's sexual essence into the partner's womb.' So, yes, yes, *yes*, according to these blokes have an orgasm ladies (no pressure!) but only *after* he climaxes or spectacularly *simultaneously* (noooooo pressure). Is that my head exploding … ?

> 'I have a low sex drive and I'm past the 'this is fun' stage so my doctor advised we do ovulation tracking. Thank goodness.' **Jane, 31**

Spiritual conception

Some of us wonder what our child might be like if the sex conceiving it was anything to go by. I remember a TTC friend of mine lamenting her child was going to be the most apathetic, frustrating little bugger imaginable thanks to their less-than-dynamic sex sessions that month. The good news is, it doesn't matter how you get the egg and the gizz together, only that they connect and set up camp in your uterus. Now, I have read a book that suggests conception is the very start of your baby's spiritual journey so you'd better honour that by making love in a welcoming, loving and spiritual way. I say screw that. Enjoy it of course, but if you don't feel like lighting candles, lovingly smiling at each other and having a simultaneous orgasm, then screw it, just do it. And then do it again the next morning!

‘Oh my God, the things I have done in bed to make it all go faster during ovulation!! My husband loved O Week – it was like Christmas.’

Anne, 29

Soldier-on sex

What's love got to do with it? Well, not much when you need to have sex again and neither of you feel like it. Alas, there's no other way of getting pregnant without some bump and grind. And there's no getting out of it. A TTC friend of mine's husband calls occasions like this ‘soldier-on sex’. It's not about love or fun, it's about duty. It's a calling, a conscription to the cause. There's no time to resent each other and focus on who signed who up for the mission. You're both in this together, soldier. Lock and load.

‘I used to dread the pressure around ovulation to have good sex or even okay sex, because there's just so much sex to have in that week and I don't always want it! To be honest neither does he. It's sometimes an absolute chore to have to get naked and turn each other on. Now we don't care if it's really bad or not, we just get it over and done with in the missionary position. We don't care about romance any more.’ **Holly, 34**

We're starting to turn each other *off*

Oh no. The sex is so bad it's not even sexy any more. TTC sex can feel mechanical, practical and about as close to 'making love' as flossing your molars. Do you stop? Do you keep going? Do you burst out laughing, claim it to be the worst TTC sex of your lives and promise to try again a few hours later? All of the above? Whatever you do, don't blame your partner for the lack of spark – you're the one who kicked off proceedings with 'I'm ovulating – let's do it' with a mouthful of toothpaste, right? Try to be encouraging, offer to do something saucy, be daring, be *sexy* – it's ovulation week!

Sex trooper tips

- Change positions.
- Stop looking so serious!
- Get the sperm-friendly lubrication out – PreSeed is a good one.
- Drag out your 'special occasions' underwear.
- Stop looking like you're … counting?
- Throw in a high voltage, spine chilling 'orgasm'!

Interruptions

There is nothing more important than bump and grind when you are TTC but life has a way of interrupting even the most militant sex schedule. Here are some tips for when you have to do it – no matter what.

When you have houseguests and it's ovulation day

Some clever planning and elaborate lying might be the only way around this one. Is it possible to plan *not* to have anyone to stay at your house during the Fertile Window? If pressed, perhaps you are having the carpets cleaned, the place needs to be fumigated or your puppy has started pooping in the spare room … If you absolutely can't get out of houseguests or simply forgot they'd be coming to stay during that all-important week, you have to – deep breath – do it anyway. Guaranteed this is not going to be the best TTC sex ever but you'll both get through it. Do it on the floor if your bed is squeaky and a poor unsuspecting relative is sleeping in the next room. Cover yourselves under the duvet and be quiet, very, very quiet. Don't worry, it'll be a funny story later. Actually, no-one wants to hear that funny story. It'll be a secret that you keep forever.

> 'I made my husband have sex with me in the car on our way to an event because I was ovulating and I knew we wouldn't be able to do it later that night. He reckons he felt 21 again but we both agreed afterwards that we're too old for that funny business!' **Karen, 38**

He's leaving on a business trip and it's ovulation day

Your partner's flight is at 6 a.m.? Do it at 4 a.m. If you know he'll be away that week, can you organise to skip out of your own work and join him on the trip? Not quite? What about flying that night to meet him? Don't go for the whole trip but a night and a morning? Can he cancel this one and stay home? Delegate it to someone else at work to take his place? Just this once? Okay, maybe again in a month's time …

> 'My husband is away a lot for work so we often do it at 4 a.m. before he has to leave – I'm half asleep when he gets started. It's definitely not the best sex!' **Karen, 38**

You have an important presentation at work during the Fertile Window

Yes, you *can* sprog up and nail that account in the same week, Supermum-To-Be. Baby-making comes first because if you feel like you didn't nail *that* – so to speak – you'll beat yourself up in the Two Week Wait and won't be able to concentrate on work anyway.

Work must be shuffled around, er, *liaising* and *workshopping* with your husband. That might mean going home at lunchtime and 'working' from home in the afternoon. It might mean doing it at 5 a.m. before your busy day starts. It might be about asking your partner to clear his work schedule and be on stand-by for the minute you get a chance to leave the office. No-one said this was going to be easy but *you* can be. You can be very, *very* easy.

> 'I just packed up and left work early one day when I got an unexpected extra line in an OPK. Nothing was stopping me being with my man!'
>
> **Sam, 33**

Desperate TTC-style seduction talk

'I'll do everything.'

'I'll do anything!'

'Please! We just have to do it! Shut up!'

PS: Your sex life will go back to being spontaneous and fun after you have had the baby. I promise!
PPS: The above is a lie, of course.

N

N is for nasty thoughts

As sweet as we are, the TTC community has some pretty nasty thoughts sometimes and I'm not talking about nasty in the American sense of the word (as in *dirty*). I'm talking about grouchy, unpleasant, mean thoughts. We *want* to be happy for the latest Smug Fertility Goddess to – oops – get pregnant while using her husband's power drill, but

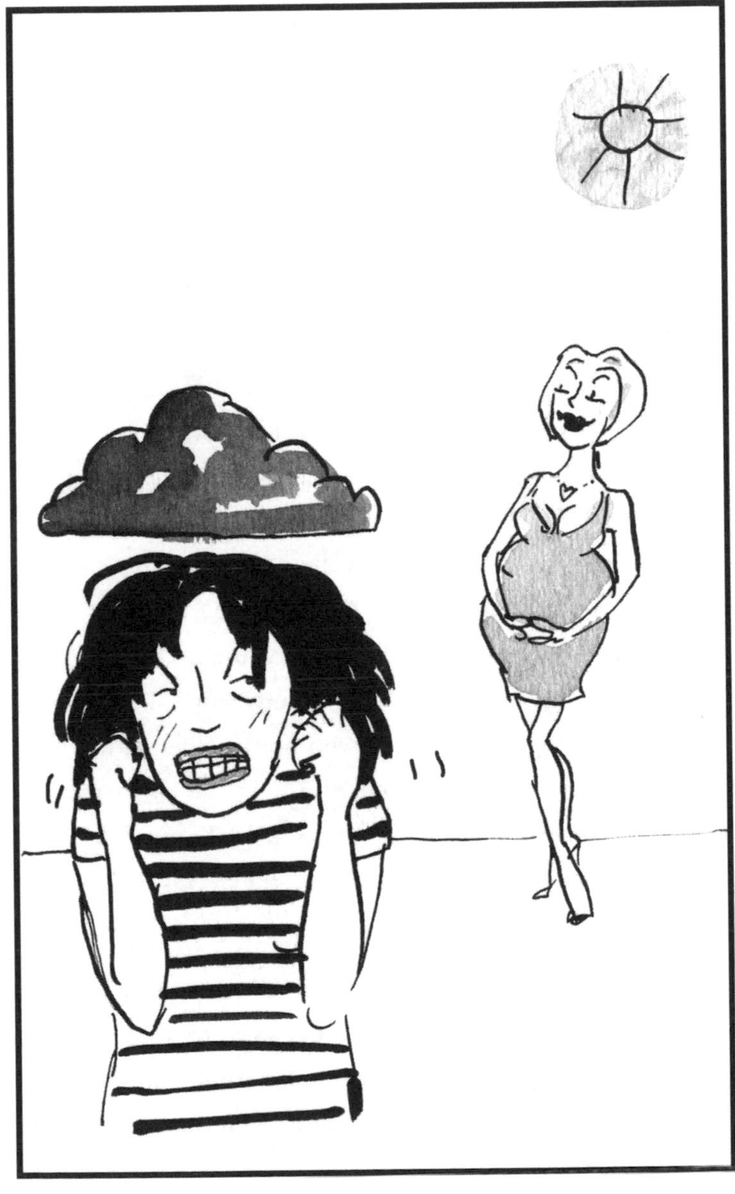

something unspeakable forces us to mutter under our breath 'Ungrateful fat cow, she already has a two-year-old!' at the news. 'It's not fair! Nothing is fair! Why her and not me? I hate her! I hope her baby is ugly!'

Nasty.

Quick Quiz: Are you consumed with nasty thoughts?

1. Instead of being pleased for the latest Smug Fertility Goddess who's parading her infant around at work, do you secretly hope the baby throws up on the boss?
2. When a friend announces she is pregnant do you secretly hope it gets her husband's big nose?
3. When your mother calls to tell you about her friend's grandchild do you secretly hope she knits it the horrid lime green bonnet she made for her last friend's grandchild?
4. Do you go out of your way to make Smug Fertility Goddesses feel as if all they do is breastfeed and hang around the house?

If you answered 'yes' to most of the above then I'm afraid you're consumed with enough inner rage to make it onto Jeremy Kyle. If you answered mostly 'no' then you are a kind and generous human being! Let's hope you bring out your 'nasty' side in the bedroom.

Instead of unleashing nasty thoughts on your partner, who doesn't have the same stress as us (although undoubtedly he does share the TTC anxiety), it might be time to vent on paper. List everything that is annoying and worrying you about TTC. And I mean everything. To get you started, here's my agro list.

Why I hate TTC:

- My cycle is so long (34 days!).
- I'm a green-eyed monster around pregnant women.
- Nothing is working.
- TTC is all I can think about.
- I'm running out of time!
- This is never going to happen for us.
- I'm not healthy enough.

And my not-so-agro list …

- My cycle is what it is (so Zen!).
- I will try to be happy for pregnant women knowing I'm going to be one of them – soon!
- I haven't tried everything – something will work.
- I must not let TTC take over my life.
- I'm only 35 (not exactly menopausal).
- I am going to stop being scared and try to be stronger.
- I will stop drinking coffee this month.

Now write down your own 'Why I hate TTC' list – along with a not-so-agro list.

> ‘I found that if the emotions running through me were anger, hopelessness, blame and sadness then that's what I'd generally get. Negativity is just a stress on the body, not just in TTC but everything.’ **Holly, 34**

Does my husband think I'm a bitch?

No! But he doesn't know exactly how you feel, no matter how many times you explain it (or sigh at him loudly). He's not inside your body. He doesn't feel those maternal instincts or the longing you feel to grow a baby inside you. Step outside yourself for a second and realise that he has to live with you too. And if he doesn't seem to want to understand, then change your approach in discussing it with him. Men tend to switch off emotionally or switch their defences on when they feel an intense or stressful conversation coming on.

Nasty thoughts about hubby

While he might not think you're a bitch, pretty soon you can't help but look at the sperm dispenser, sorry, your husband, and think ‘Maybe it's him and all the coffee/beer/tight undies.’ It can get mean. TTC can be one big incredibly frustrating unanswered question and then about a million little questions inside it. Is it you? Is it me? Is it all in my head?

Is it the ciggies he smoked last month at a party? Is it the coffee he can't give up? Is it those damned tight undies he wears to bed? Or, oh no, is it that we just don't *work* together? Hmm. It's easy to blame the one you love. Don't. Or at least try not to.

> 'I've never been so confronted by my own bleak mood than when TTC but you just have to know that it changes – and fast. It's hard but it's important to know that this feeling is *not* going to last.' **Cath, 34**

Is it because I'm so bitter and nasty that I don't deserve a baby?

Noooooo! You're stressed, under pressure and this is taking longer than you thought it might. You're a good person, you deserve a baby. Keep reminding yourself of that. And give yourself a break.

> 'The year we were TTC I was a bitch most of the time, I couldn't help it, and I didn't care after a while. I just felt sad and disappointed and under pressure all the time. I just couldn't take anything lightly. I remember laughing one day and thinking 'God, I haven't laughed in ages.' It's important to laugh!' **Heather, 36**

Why am I so f***ing angry?

Because this feels out of control, TTC isn't fair and the Baby Gods suck. It is totally understandable that you feel angry – we all do! But it might be more fun being active instead. Go for a walk. Turn up the music and dance. Shake your body out all over. Jump up and down. Or try one of these suggestions:

Goodbye nasty thoughts

- Take time out for yourself every day.
- Put your feet up and zone out – stop thinking!
- Record negative emotions in the Bump & Grind diary (better out than in).
- Stick a few affirmations to your fridge or bathroom mirror.
- Chant positive words and phrases in your head like 'healthy', 'happy' and 'sexy yummy mummy in the making'.
- Have sex on non-fertile days just for fun.
- Eliminate negativity around you.
- Don't hang out with negative, angry people.
- Don't let yourself be dragged into conflict.
- Say 'no' when you need to keep personal boundaries.
- Put yourself first.
- Choose to be happy.

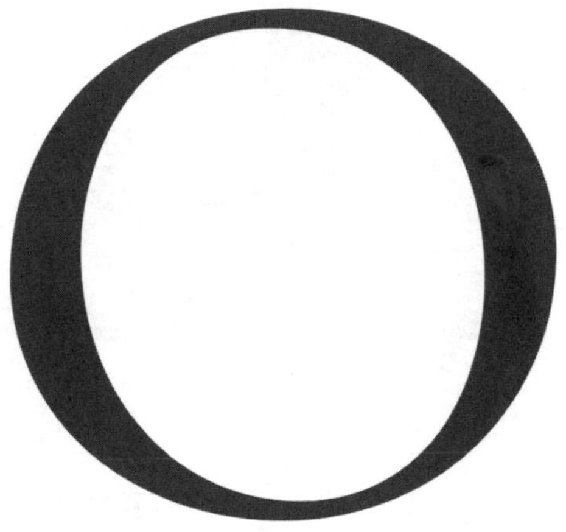

O is for Oprah

O is for *what now, girlfriend*? O is for Oprah. It's a silly chapter title, I know, but some women, lots of successful women – like gal pal Oprah – don't have babies. What if you didn't have a baby of your own? Would you adopt a baby? Would you throw yourself into your relationship or your career and become one of those cute couples who are stand-out favourite

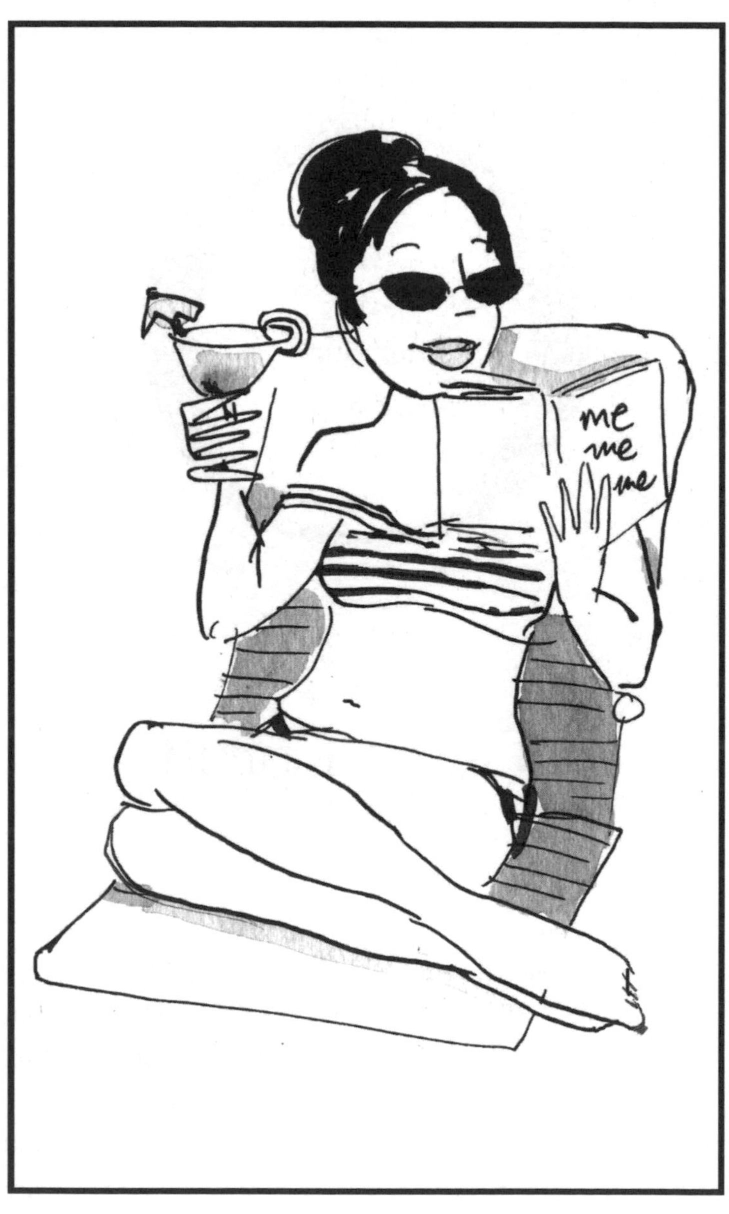
me
me
me

aunts and uncles and spoil their nieces and nephews? Meanwhile they travel, have fabulous relationships without tedious TTC sex, and they enjoy each other – just the way they are. It's not such a bad thought. It's a really nice thought! And it's good to put things into perspective once in a while. Here's a little more of that …

Brutal witching hour cheer up

Sometime soon, book a date with an especially busy mum you know and just spend time with her 'helping out with the kids' between 4 p.m. and 7 p.m. – the witching hour. The witching hour (which most parents will tell you can last up to five hours) is where children have 'hit their limit' of niceness for the day and become a *tad* unreasonable. Your friend's children might be ratty, demanding, perhaps falling on the floor in tears while screaming at their poor frazzled mum (who could do with another vino). They might be throwing their dinner on the ground – the dinner their poor tired mum spent half an hour making while simultaneously hanging out the laundry, mopping vomit off the couch and raking a comb through her hair (which has formed dreadlocks underneath from the use of time-saving two-in-one shampoo and conditioner). If that doesn't make you race home feeling just as glad as glad can be that you *currently* don't have a baby then nothing will. Phew!

How to celebrate *not* having a baby (yet)

Have a look around. See anything with baby poop/vomit/drool on it? Can you talk to your partner without having to shriek over a wailing infant? Can you race out the door to get to a shoe sale, a yoga class or just leave the room for five minutes before you throw yourself on the floor in a crying heap (as many new mums would like to!). Enjoy this time friends, because everything changes. This TTC phase just isn't going to last. You *are* going to have a baby and you'll be knee deep in nappies mourning your former life soon enough. Love and cherish your space, your body, your home and your partner – just the way they are!

> 'Every now and then when I'm feeling selfish and loving my own time and company I just go 'phew'.' **Anne, 29**

The good life

Savour the life you have now by indulging in some of the following.

- Go out for dinner and get a little tipsy.
- Sleep in.
- Read all the weekend papers in bed.
- Call a friend with children and note how many times she is interrupted to scream 'Please! Give me a minute on the phone!'
- Consider turning your future baby room into a

study or 'play' room (you can always change it back again!).

- Go see a movie.
- Spend a whole Sunday reading a book.
- Plan a trip away.
- Cuddle your dog.
- Have a bath with a luscious bath bomb and big glass of wine.
- Turn the music up.
- Talk about a five-year plan with your partner – and how much money you'll have!
- Put all your TTC books (not this one!) at the back of your closet.
- Go out with your single friends and listen to their dating tales.
- Cuddle your partner, be grateful for your life together.

'We spend lots of time with couples who don't have children yet or who have made the decision to not have children at all. They think all our efforts to conceive are hilarious – they're just happy with their life together! What a relief it must be to feel that way.' **Kate, 28**

Me Time versus Mummyville

Where did it all the Me Time go? When you have a new baby Me Time gets snatched somewhere between a two-minute shower at midnight and staring at a teleshopping channel on TV at 4 a.m. while breastfeeding on the couch. New baby joy aside, it can be depressing. When I was hard-core TTC a frazzled new mum friend of mine worked very *hard* to let me know just how lucky I was to be *sans* infant. She used to growl at me 'Enjoy it, enjoy it, *enjoy* it! You still have a life!' And she was right. So, let's compare shall we? Just for the sake of feeling good about not having a baby (yet).

An ordinary Saturday without a baby

3 a.m.: You're asleep, of course!

9 a.m.: Wake up and kiss your partner, note the time and exclaim 'What a great lie-in!'

10 a.m.: Venture out for breakfast together to your favourite café, picking up the weekend papers on the way. Note how fit you look in a shop window while walking by – nice butt!

1 p.m.: Go for a walk with a girlfriend and talk about work, a new project you are embarking on and how much you're looking forward to watching the finale of *Britain's Got Talent.*

3 p.m.: Read a book in the sun, take a nap, pull out a few weeds in the garden.

6 p.m.: Start making a fancy dinner for you, your partner and some close friends, pop the champers early.
11 p.m.: Fall into bed.

An ordinary Saturday *with* a new baby

3 a.m.: Breastfeed.
9 a.m.: Breastfeed while nagging your husband over the dirty washing that's piling up on your bed.
10 a.m.: Breastfeed while wondering if you're ever going to shower again, if you have nipple thrush, why you still look eight months pregnant and if your boobs will ever go back to anything other than a droopy D-cup.
1 p.m.: Breastfeed while reading up on 'hysterical fits of crying all through the night'.
3 p.m.: Breastfeed while wondering how you can balance the baby while looking out the lounge room window to the outside world.
6 p.m.: Breastfeed while waiting for your dinner to defrost in the microwave.
11 p.m.: Breastfeed while sleeping upright on the couch.

Yep, that's generally how it goes. But you knew all that, right? And you still want it ... Well, *maybe*. Wanting a baby is *wanting a baby* no matter how hard you know it's going to be and how long you'll still be wearing maternity pants afterwards … but it *is* nice to step out of the TTC world just long enough to see how good your life is – just the way it is.

> ‘I have to accept that I might lose this one. And that's okay. I can't win at everything. I don't have to be cheerful about it but I have to accept it somehow, and that makes it a bit easier.’ **Barb, 36**

> ‘Everyone deals with something in life and I have to be grateful for what I already have. A friend of mine has two kids and was recently diagnosed with breast cancer. Life is hard for everyone in some way.’ **Sal, 31**

PS: One day Ben and I sat down together and asked if we'd be happy without a baby of our own and the answer – after some thought – was 'Yes'. It's a biggie. But it might be worth asking.

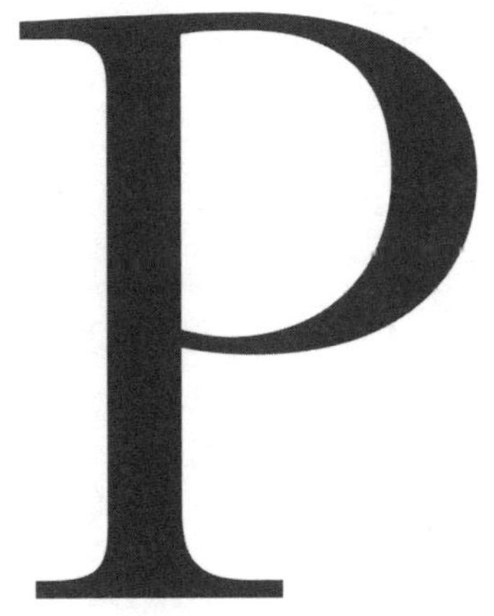

P is for period party

Bloody hell, not your period again. And now it's time to *party*? Yes. Not party as in splurging on drugs and alcohol (although that will remove the pain for a night or two) but party as in set aside some time and money to do whatever you want. Whatever makes you feel good. Whatever cheers you up. In other words, from now on your period

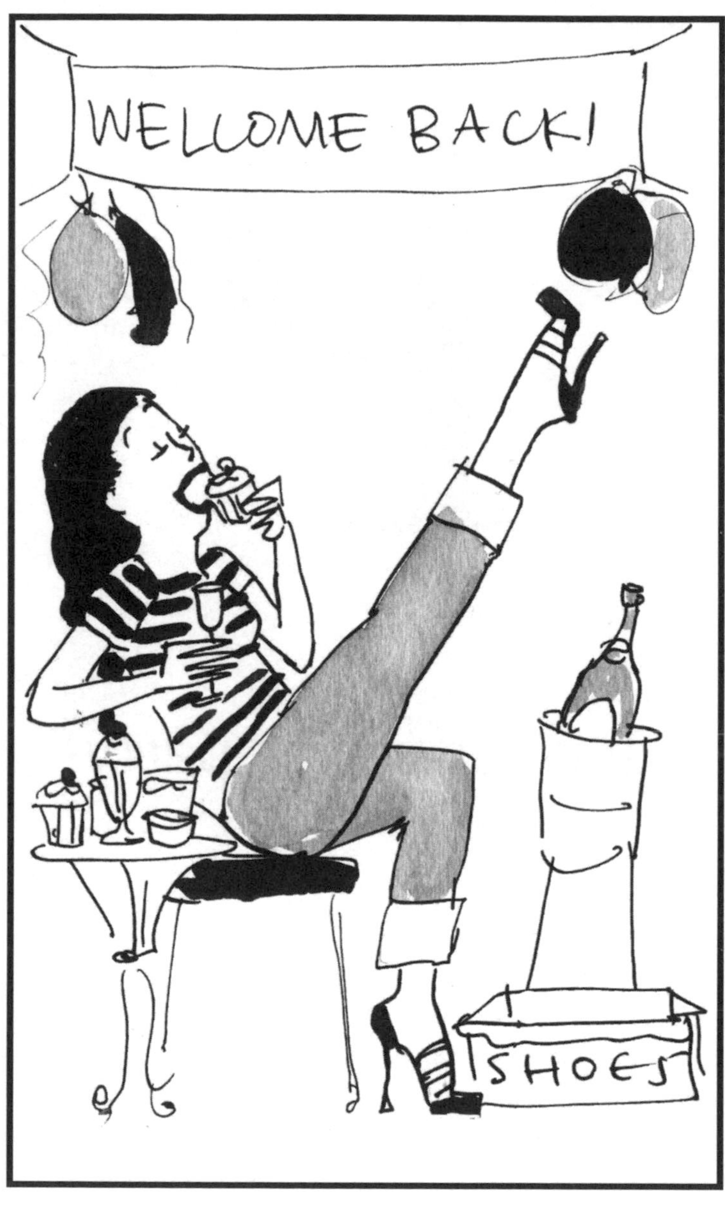
WELCOME BACK!
SHOES

doesn't have to be a super-absorbent maxi pad bummer (with wings).

A TTC friend of mine loves pigging out on fancy brie cheese and would allow herself half a wheel (!) of the really good stuff with a big glass of red wine when she got her period. Another would buy herself a new outfit every time 'Aunt Flo' came to town. For me it's always buying new pyjamas and having a night alone on the couch to watch shamelessly tacky television.

> 'Aunt Flo is a witch, sorry, make that a bitch.'
>
> **Heather, 36**

Period party favourites:

- Break out the comfort food.
- Rent all the feel-good movies you like and watch them all weekend.
- Buy new shoes, lots of new shoes.
- Spend an uninterrupted night on the couch fondling the remote control.
- Book in for a facial.
- Buy yourself ridiculously pricey appliances for the kitchen.
- Allow yourself to cry, cry, cry, if you want to.
- Have a weekend *all* to yourself to potter around the house – don't answer the phone, switch off your mobile.

- Take your partner out for breakfast.
- Book a mini break and just get away from your town and your everyday life.

Period pick-me-up

This is a bit icky but one of the Fertility Sisters helped me look at my period a bit differently when I told her that getting it every month when we were TTC made me angry and depressed.

'No, no, no!' she said. 'Your period is what makes you a woman, makes you fertile, your period is what's going to make having a baby possible! You want a lot of blood, a good lining, healthy new blood, enjoy the blood!'

Hmm. Enjoy the blood?

I'm not sure about that. But we are going to give a shout out to the hormones that make having a baby possible every month.

Hallelujah hormones

Good reproductive health is when a nice balance between the hormones regulates the events that make up each cycle. Let's take a look at those hormones one by one.

Oestrogen: This hormone promotes the development and maintenance of female reproductive structures (especially the endometrial lining of the uterus). It also assists in the control of fluid and electrolyte balance within the body, and prepares the follicle for the release of an egg.

Progesterone: This hormone helps to prepare the endometrium (womb lining) for the implantation of an egg.

Follicle stimulating hormone (FSH): FSH stimulates the follicles to ripen several eggs.

Lutenising hormone (LH): Triggers ovulation. Certain lifestyle factors will all help regulate your hormones: your diet, not binging on alcohol, staying Zen and getting at least eight hours sleep a night. And for now, your period is just part of that amazing process.

And, if you want to go right over the top in loving Aunt Flo, according to naturopathic and homeopathic physician Dr Judyth Reichenberg-Ullman: 'Your menstrual cycle is a beautiful outpouring of your feminine nature and spirit. Love and appreciate this aspect of your life as a symbol of the overall flow and outpouring of your life.'

PS: Hmm. That's just a bit weird.

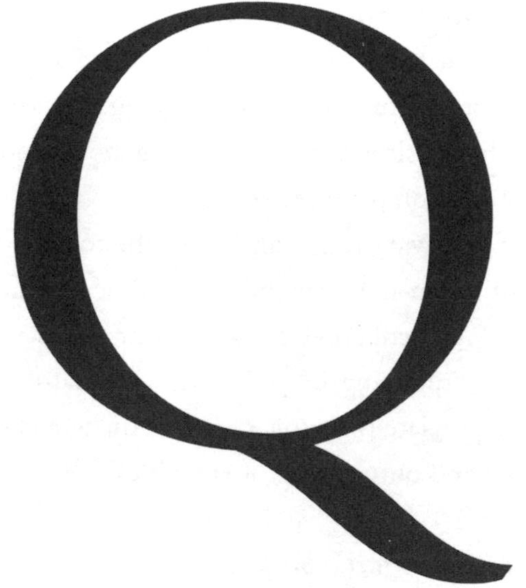

Q is for quitting TTC

Put down the thermometer and step away from your chart. You're so addicted to TTC you don't do calendar dates – you do cycle days. And you've gone from being 'just good friends' with your cervix to something much, much deeper …

We all get a little addicted to TTC. It's all the planning, the hoping and the perpetual thought 'This could be the

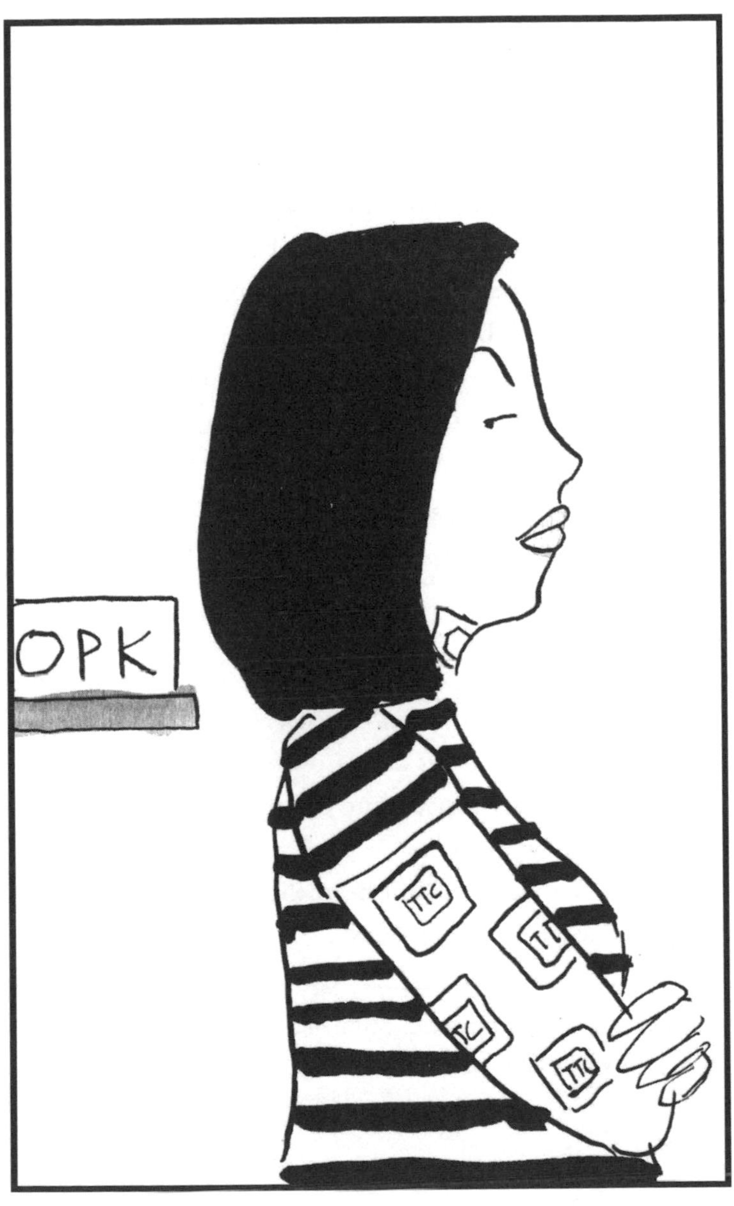
OPK
TTC
TTC

month!' But sometimes the thought of not poking about your cervix and pumping yourself with supplements seems really, really appealing.

A TTC friend of mine tells me she felt 'broken' after a year of TTC. She said while IVF may solve her baby problems, something had indelibly changed in her and she needed to mend it first. I felt that way too. Before I 'hopped' on the Way of The Bunny Rabbit to get pregnant (read on) I had to step out of the TTC routine and find myself again, or at least get a glimpse of her. Most blame the Two Week Wait for wanting to quit because it can be such a roller-coaster of emotions. The idea of simply getting out of your carriage and walking away is very, very tempting. But is it enough to quit?

It might be time to quit when:

- you feel 'broken'
- you feel as if you've lost yourself
- you feel as if TTC is taking over your relationship
- you can barely concentrate on anything else, especially your job
- you know deep in your heart that all the stress might be preventing a pregnancy.

> 'Obsessed, obsessed, obsessed. To just be myself again would be nice. If I could go back ...' **Jane, 31**

Am I just 'giving up' to fool myself into getting pregnant?

Haven't we all tried to play hard to get with the Baby Gods? If I say I don't want it – then I might get it? Ben and I 'gave up' in the month we conceived in that we ditched our impossibly organised sex routine and I went back to doing all the things I used to love before TTC, like yoga, and spending time with my girlfriends. But I'm sure, at the back of our minds, we were still hoping that our new 'Zen' approach might just work. And that's okay. You don't have to be *officially* one or the other – trying or not trying. It's all about taking the pressure off and not being so hard on yourself.

Perhaps instead of quitting the whole thing completely, you could stop charting your temperature, or stop having sex when you 'think you should' and do it every other day. You could stop talking about it for a month. Ben and I had talked about it so much for 18 months that in the month we conceived we had made a pact with each other (well, I'd promised to zip it!) to not talk about TTC and just live our lives. The best thing about a break is that it can give you some breathing space to remember who you were before TTC and enjoy each other again.

> 'I couldn't give up TTC if I tried. I just know my cycle too well – without even looking at my chart I know exactly what's going on. As if I could just pretend I wasn't thinking about that and planning to have sex on that day. If only!'
>
> **Hannah, 31**

Project or problem?

The thrill of getting a smiley face on a digital OPK or when your period is a day late! It's an irresistible mix of anticipation and hope that's hard to let go of; it's almost impossible sometimes. Plus, what if you give up and miss ovulation completely? That's another month gone! It can all be addictive. You just have to ask yourself how much your TTC addiction is taking over your life and if it's still a project or a full-blown problem.

Quick Quiz: Are you addicted to TTC?

1. Are you more intimate with your BBT chart than your husband?
2. Do you buy pregnancy tests in bulk over the Internet?
3. Does the thought of *not* taking your temperature each morning fill you with panic?
4. Have you ever spent an entire afternoon at work Googling pregnancy signs and symptoms?
5. Does the thought of missing ovulation this month fill you with more anxiety than missing your dad's 60th birthday party?

If you answered 'yes' to most of the above then it might be time for a stint in TTC rehab or at least a patch or two. If you answered 'no' to most of the above then you're still a 'social' TTC-er and you only obsess at certain times of the month, you can quit any time you like …

'I once lost my thermometer and I was an hour late for work looking for it while crying hysterically and blaming my husband for moving it. I would have kept searching *all* day. My husband found it under our bed, he wasn't happy.' **Cath, 34**

How to cut back

- Stop taking your temperature every morning.
- Try a month without talking about TTC with your partner.
- Don't use both urine and saliva ovulation tests – just pick one.
- Promise yourself not to obsess about every little twinge in the Two Week Wait and plan a long weekend escape instead.
- Explore a few new interests that have nothing to do with fertility management that are fun.

'I got so exhausted thinking about it all the time. I got to a point where I couldn't do it any more and I gave myself permission to stop. I don't think that helped me get pregnant, but it made me feel better.' **Donna, 36**

PS: We all have our TTC vices. Mine is analysing the 'ferning' patterns in my saliva ovulation microscope so curiously I could be a forensic scientist. Hmm, maybe there's a support group for that …

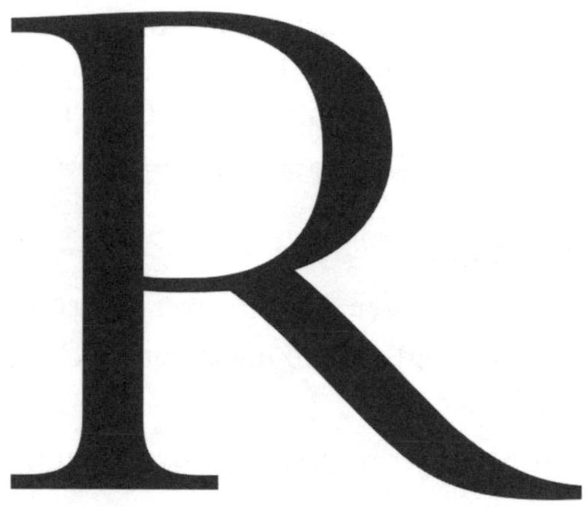

R is for rela– don't say it!

There is only one swear word in the TTC world – 'relax'! Ugh, I can feel a shudder among you, fists clenched, lips pursed. There's no denying there is nothing more irksome to the TTC community than when someone suggests that we relax in order to get pregnant. As if that's the secret. As if that's the one thing we haven't considered. As if it's as

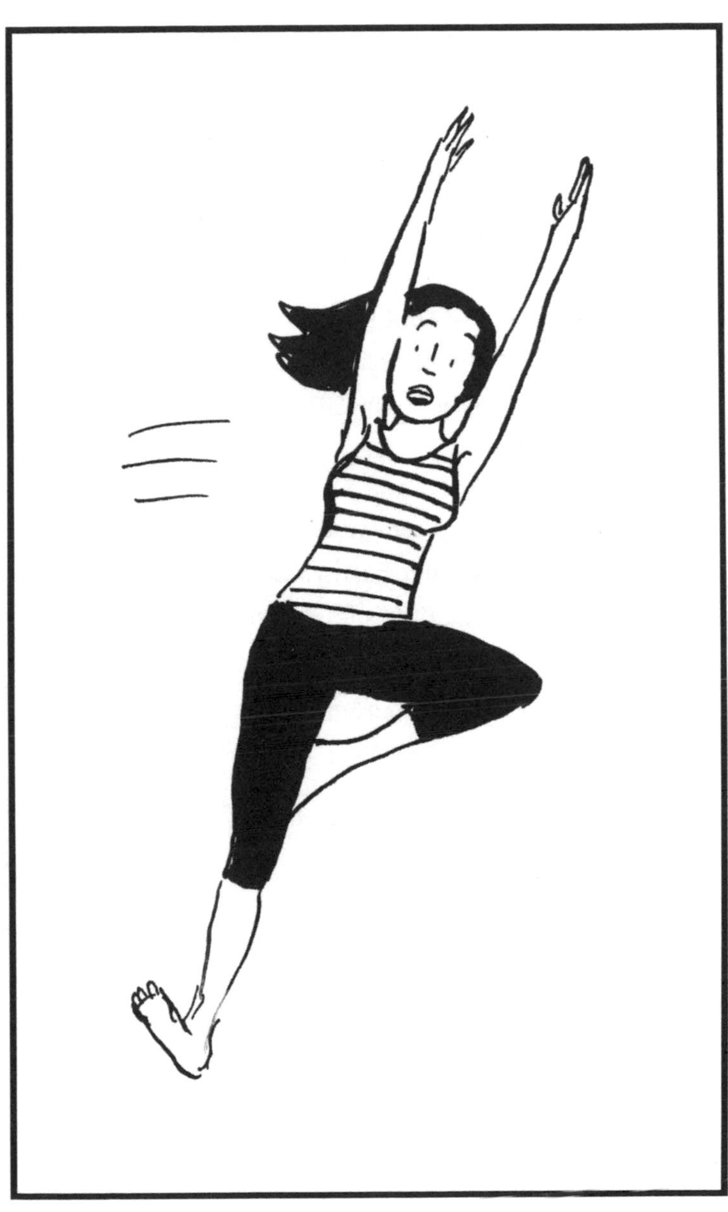

easy as that! It's a slap in the face to anyone who has had the stress of trying to have a baby when all around you women are popping out of the nappy aisle at the supermarket with 'Guess what? I'm pregnant! Again!' Grrrrr.

How the R word makes us feel:

- as if that's the answer to all fertility problems (no amount of relaxing is going to unblock a fallopian tube or clear away endometriosis)
- that we're too uptight and strung out to join the Mummy Club
- as if it's our fault
- as if our careers are to blame
- as if we're not Mother Earthy enough
- as if we haven't thought of 'relaxing' already.

> 'It's the most insensitive and ignorant thing that someone can say to a couple struggling to conceive. I don't believe there is anything in it at all when you need treatment. I could have relaxed until I was dead and still not fallen pregnant.'
>
> **Kim, 37**

Why do people tell us to 'relax'?

- Because they are clueless as to how much time it can take and how hard it can be to get pregnant.
- Because it's easy advice to give without really thinking.

- Because they sense we are under pressure and want us to calm down.
- Because they're not used to seeing us upset.
- Because some annoying Smug Fertility Goddess once swore that was all it took.

What to say when someone says 'Just relax and you'll get pregnant!'

'Good idea! Let's meditate together! I'll go get my mat.'

'It's weird but people *telling* me to relax just makes me psychotic.'

'I'm not sure if relaxing will unblock a fallopian tube/clear away endometriosis or remove a cyst from an ovary – but thanks!'

'I *was* relaxed ... until we started talking.'

'I'm not sure there's anything in that "relax" crap ... cup of tea?'

'Oh, I think really uptight women get pregnant too ... how many kids do you have?'

The truth is our bodies weren't designed to get pregnant under a certain amount of stress or anxiety. Back in the day you might not have gotten pregnant running from a sabre-toothed tiger. And today, you might not get pregnant when you have job stress, money stress, emotional stress, negative thinking or unhealthy lifestyle stress on your body. When TTC becomes stressful too, the body recognises that as a 'fight or flight' situation and reacts accordingly.

'Lots of women find it impossible to still themselves – it's way too much of a challenge. To express and have validated the myriad feelings that arise when conception is challenging, I believe, is a vital first step towards a still mind.' **Fertility acupuncturist and Chinese herbalist, Shauna Cason**

Me, stressed?

When the Fertility Sisters told me the only way I would get pregnant was to stop *thinking* so much and yep, *relax*, I rang my sister in tears. 'I'm not sure if I've relaxed in a year!' I sobbed, 'What do they meeeean?' She promised to send me soothing hippie music and lavender oil to burn.

I was clueless. Relax? Like, sit down and stop thinking? Go for a walk? I honestly wasn't exactly sure what true 'relaxing' might entail. And regardless, wasn't I a pretty relaxed person in the big picture anyway? Then I realised that I was spending a portion of my work days sort of holding my breath and scowling at the phone. I was rushing to meet deadlines and spending a chunk of my time tearing my hair out when things didn't go to plan. Not to mention the almost daily upsets that TTC would bring to any work day. Add to that the sleepless nights I spent worrying where all the TTC was going …

Maybe I *was* stressed … Are you?

What exactly is a 'relaxed' state?

Most people relax on holidays. Other people feel relaxed when they escape their everyday lives through books, movies or half a bottle of chardonnay on a Saturday night. Lots of people relax when they are most active – either power-walking through the park or tearing up their garden. Some people call this a 'moving meditation', where your body is active but your mind is at peace. Everyone is different. Sometimes it's just the company of certain people that makes us chill out. Sometimes we only ever truly get it when we are alone.

Here's what it might feel like for you …

- there's a quietness in your mind (no chatter of negative thoughts or just 'busy brain')
- there's a sense of balance, things are just right
- there's no tightness in your shoulders, back or face
- you have a sense of letting go
- there's a feeling time has slowed down or is right in the moment, with you, not racing ahead without you
- you possess a feeling of contentment for yourself and those around you
- you're in an unworried and unhurried state
- you're in a sort of comfortable limbo of not feeling high or low – just sitting comfortably somewhere in the middle.

> 'Just telling women to relax is ridiculous; you have to offer them insight into what it really feels like. Some women may never have felt truly relaxed.'
>
> **Fertility acupuncturist and Chinese herbalist, Shauna Cason**

The effects of stress on fertility

In technical terms, stress can affect the functioning of the hypothalamus. This is the gland in the brain that regulates not only appetite and emotions but the hormones required to release the eggs in women and produce sperm in men. When you are really stressed, you may ovulate much later in your cycle or not at all. To go back to the very beginning, it's like when the Fertility Sisters told me that if I was a bunny rabbit the message I was sending my body was that there wasn't enough green grass around to feed little bunnies so things just shut down. Until I stopped stressing and effectively told my body there was plenty of green grass, there would be no little bunnies.

Will my body tell me if I'm too stressed?

Some women are so used to feeling slightly stressed with their work and lives in general that they ovulate pretty normally while others only need a sudden bout of stress to throw out their cycle. It varies from woman to woman. Your cervical mucus might also let you know when you are too stressed.

Instead of wetness around ovulation time you might get a few wet days then dry – as if your body is trying to ovulate but stress is delaying it.

> 'I see so many women who lead busy, stressful lives. They don't take any quiet time, they're anxious and overworked and don't sleep enough. They say they are doing everything to conceive but really, the most important thing might be just to slow down.' **Fertility acupuncturist and Chinese herbalist, Shauna Cason**

But TTC is making me stressed!

We can't get pregnant when we're really stressed but not getting pregnant is the *reason* we're really stressed! The bad news is that research does show that women going through infertility treatment (such as IVF) suffer heightened stress similar to those dealing with life-threatening illnesses such as cancer and heart disease. It's because there is so much waiting, hoping and disappointment when things don't go to plan. The most important thing to do right now might be to really look at what's making us stressed. Let's put our TTC stress in a different basket to everyday stress.

Everyday stress (mostly external): work; family; friends; commitments; busyness; money; the everyday demands we place on ourselves.

TTC stress (mostly internal): anxiety felt in the Two Week Wait; getting your period; worrying something might be wrong; worrying about tests; worrying treatment won't work; worrying about the future; waiting for results; not being able to see beyond each cycle.

What are your stressors? What makes you feel stressed? Sometimes just writing them out will help send them packing. Or just help you to see them clearly.

'When you're TTC, try not to think in the immediacy of the moment. It becomes too hard when you hang everything on if you get your period or not. Keep looking to the next cycle and the one after.'

IVF specialist, Dr Bill Watkins

The 10-step TTC chill out

1. Stop what you're doing.
2. Take a deep breath.
3. Find a comfortable, quiet place (even an office bathroom cubicle will work!).
4. Sit down.
5. Close your eyes.
6. Breathe in and out deeply, three times.
7. Make each breath a little longer and slower than the last.
8. Let your mind wander to a happy, peaceful place and imagine yourself there.

9. Simply be still in that place, let thoughts come and go, keep breathing, stay there a little while.
10. Slowly open your eyes and stretch.

'So often women will lie down on my table for acupuncture and tell me that it's the first time they've had any quiet time all week. Immediately I hear alarm bells in my head.' **Fertility acupuncturist and Chinese herbalist, Shauna Cason**

Quick Quiz: How stressed are you?

1. Do you suffer from insomnia or anxiety?
2. Do you find yourself holding your breath or taking small, shallow breaths?
3. Have you forgotten the last time you took some real time out for yourself?
4. Do you work longer and longer hours and still not feel you're on top of everything?
5. Are you quick to snap at people close to you?
6. Do you have a constant feeling of panic that you won't have a baby or that you're running out of time?

If you answered 'yes' to most of the above then forget *road* rage, you probably suffer from the odd bout of TTC rage. It might be time to stop, take a deep breath and get some balance back in your everyday life (or just take your hand off the horn). If you answered mostly 'no' then you're probably chilled out – except when people mention the R word!

> 'Do yourself a favour and stop stressing. If you're really frustrated after only trying for a few months then you're going to send yourself crazy.' **Karen, 38**

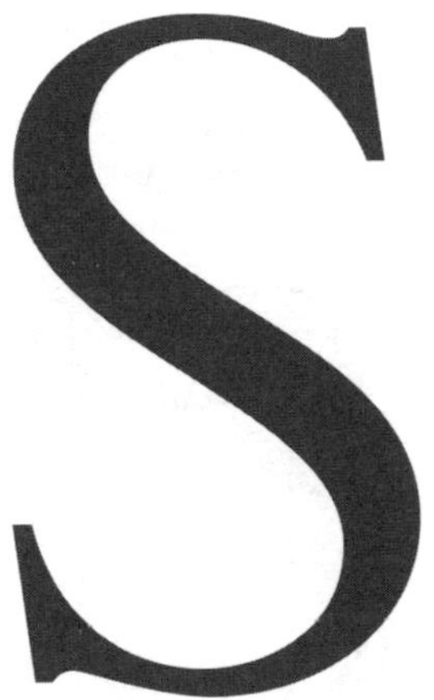

S is for Smug Fertility Goddess

Oooh, we don't like her! She's the belly-stroking super-fertile woman who smiles serenely and suggests you calm down and 'relax' in order to conceive. You probably didn't really notice her before you started trying to get pregnant. She was just the woman who always seemed to have a baby hanging from her boob and a

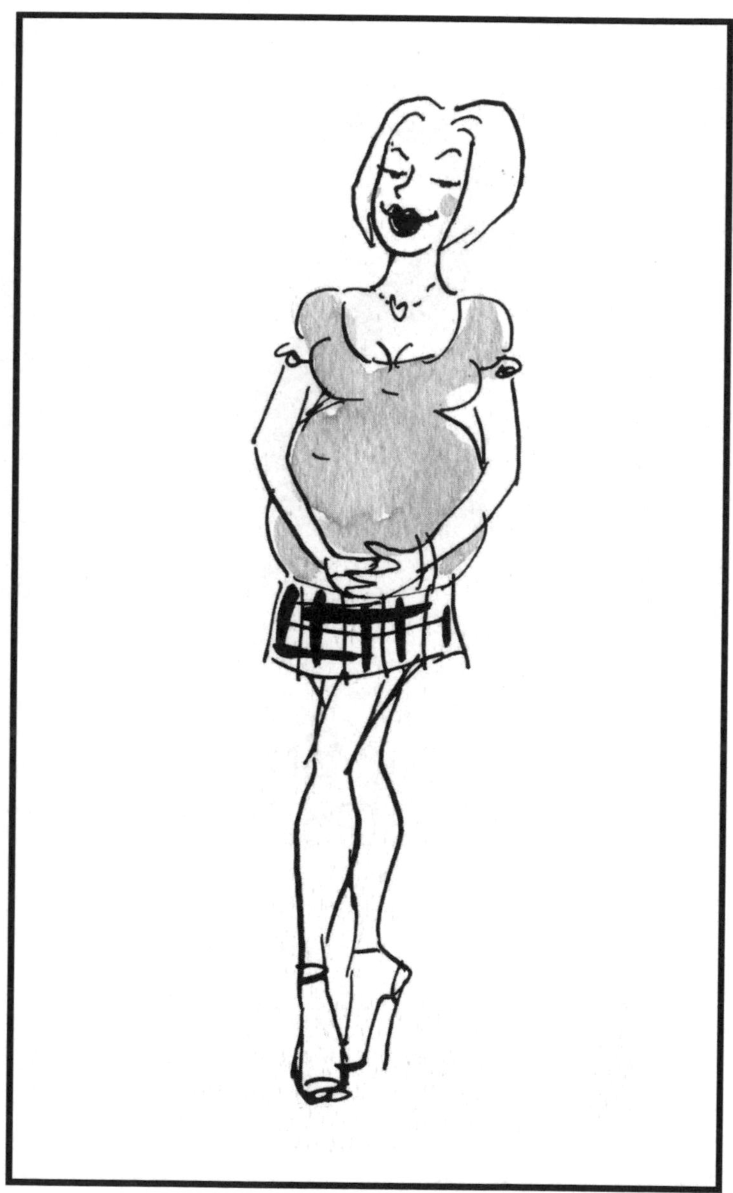

very tired-looking husband. Now she's everywhere with her cute maternity tops and prenatal yoga postures. She might even be among your best friends. Without doubt, the minute you decide to have a baby an SFG will pop out of the nappy aisle in the supermarket to make you feel bad about yourself. You can't let her.

So what is a Smug Fertility Goddess? She is:

- a woman who recklessly brags about her fertility in front of her reproductively challenged friends. She either got pregnant the first go or without really trying.
- a woman who has *no clue* what we're going through but doesn't take a moment to consider how her talk might be hurting our feelings
- a woman who makes you feel like her pregnancy is the only thing going on in the universe and somehow she is a deity for making it happen and should be worshipped while coasting around on a lily pad.

> 'The minute that pregnant women get that disgusting faraway look on their faces while rubbing their bellies, I want to puke.' **Kate, 28**

Why we don't like her

Well, to be really honest, it's because we want to *be* her – without the smug part. Any woman who has battled the Baby Gods and lived to tell the tale is never, ever smug

– even if she goes on to have five kids. It's hard to like anyone who gets the things we want too easily without a fight or at least a struggle along the way. And then goes on to brag about it.

'They act like what they're doing – gestating – is the one and only thing going on in the world. It's the centre of the universe and all they want to talk about. Arrrghh!! Shut up already!' **Sam, 33**

'I can't stand the ones who post pictures of their growing pregnant bellies on the web that they take in the mirror. And the ones who talk about nothing but their unborn child – who they've nicknamed – in their status posts on Facebook.' **Karen, 38**

Why do women brag about their fertility?

I was once at a baby shower where the mum-to-be told the gathering her hubby 'hit a six off the first ball' – as in she got pregnant on their very first try – and then she laughed smugly into her ginger tea. The groan among the TTC-ers (including me) was audible and I secretly hoped her baby would be a puker (turns out he was, hurrah!). The women who brag about how easy it was to get pregnant don't understand. That's all. They're not hurtful, stupid or completely void of sensitivity (well, most of them aren't) they just haven't spent two weeks out of every month squinting at their nipples hoping to see blue veins. They haven't stared at a home pregnancy test for 20 minutes and *begged* it to show another line. They haven't wondered what it might be like to *never* have a baby.

They simply have no idea what we're going through. Back in the day I think she called herself Fertile Myrtle. 'Oh my husband just has to look at me and I get pregnant!' Or, 'I just have to walk past my husband and I get pregnant!' Well stop standing in his way, I say!

In ancient times, fertility goddesses were the female deities who watched over and promoted fertility, pregnancy and birth in many polytheistic cultures. Those über-fertiles included Aphrodite in ancient Greece, Hathor in ancient Egypt and the Teutonic goddess Freyja. I don't think we would have liked those smug babes either.

> 'Women get pregnant all the time, it's not like you've found a cure for cancer.' **Holly, 34**

How to deal with an SFG

In order to deal with an SFG, you just have to keep a healthy sense of self at all times. Repeat after me: I am not inferior, missing the mummy gene or not a goddess just because I am not a *fertility* goddess (yet). I am Goddess of the Immaculate Ovulation Calendar. I am Goddess of the 2 p.m. Ovulation

Predictor Kit Test. I am Goddess of the Ridiculously Early Pregnancy Test. You *are* a goddess. You are a *goddess!* Don't stop believing that. The SFG in your life just got lucky quicker and easier than you, but no doubt there are areas of your life that *she* envies. Like your career, your supportive husband, your free time and your baby-vomit-free clothes. The grass might look greener over there in the baby stakes but no picture is ever perfect. Love your own patch of grass – it's pretty great!

'I hate the way Smug Pregnants smile no matter what they are talking about. They have that icky pregnant lady smile. And they're never really listening to you. [They're] just pondering the constant wonder of their unborn child. You smug bitch, wake up!' **Anne, 29**

Things to feel great about

- You'll never, ever, be smug, even when you stick it to the Baby Gods and become that glowing fertility goddess you want to be – and not being smug is a really nice thing!
- When you do get pregnant – and that's going to be soon! – you're going to enjoy it even more than your average SFG.
- You're much closer to your partner thanks to the TTC experience.

- The time you've already spent TTC means you'll never do that time again – you're months closer to your goal!

'Smug pregnant women get this look: 'It's all meaningless, nothing is as wondrous as me and my unborn child.' I always hope her breasts go *really* floppy and her little miracle will be spewing on her soon enough. Ha!' **Hannah, 31**

PS: Not all women who get pregnant really easily are Smug Fertility Goddesses. There are lots of women who just happen to be Super Fertiles and they don't bang on about it. We like them. In fact, rub yourself against one of those blessed babes for extra good luck.

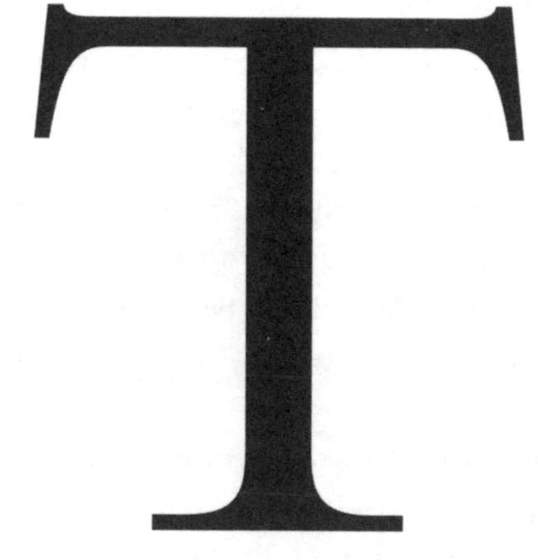

T is for the Two Week Wait

The Two Week Wait: the best of times, the worst of times. A time when stubbing your toe can be a sign of pregnancy, or absolute confirmation otherwise. It's a time of great hope and despair. Hope that *this could be the month!* And despair, *oh God, what if it's not?* Most of us obsess about every little twinge in our bodies: if our boobs are

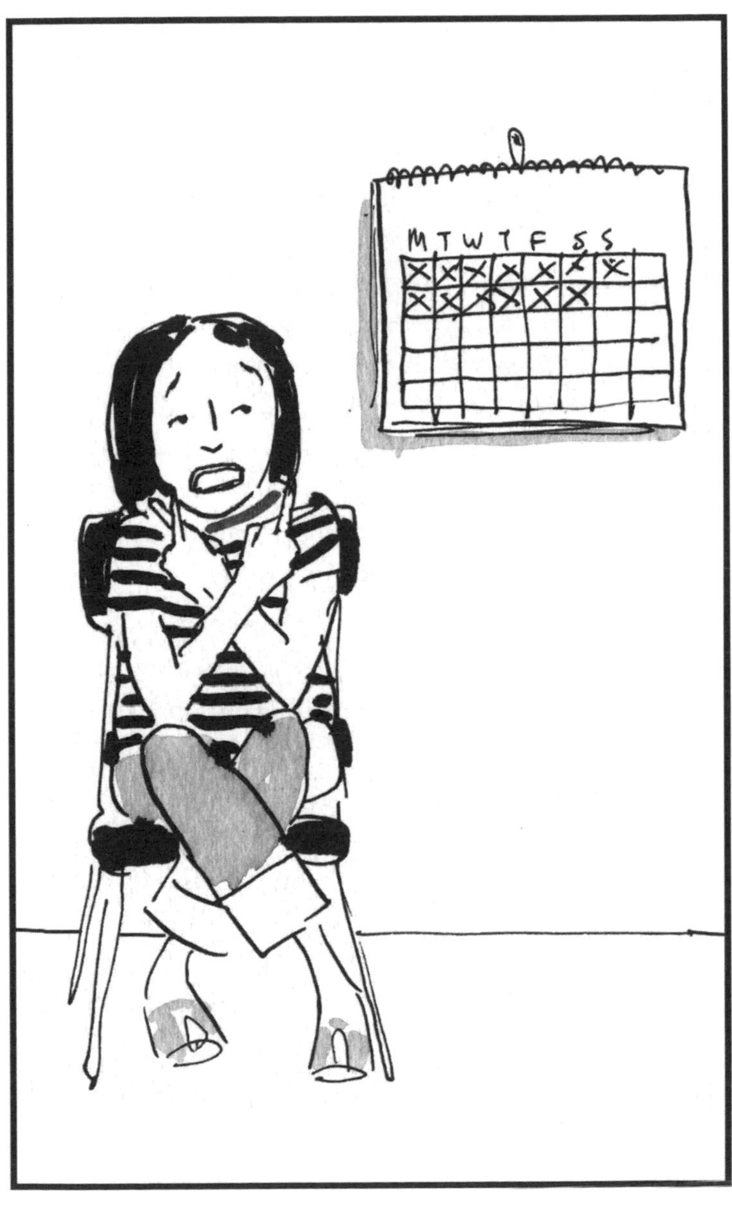
M T W T F S S

tingly or achy, if we feel a headache coming on or if it's just from staring too long and hard at our nipples in the mirror looking for pretty blue veins. The month Ben and I conceived was the month I felt the fewest number of signs and symptoms but there were definite little things that made me think 'this just might be it'. The biggest indication was I spent the first week of the Two Week Wait in tears and the second week being an emotional lunatic. Ben *carefully* suggested something just had to be up …

The Two Week Wait is the greatest roller-coaster in TTC – which means you're allowed to close your eyes and scream a little here and there. For now, let's obsess and then obsess some more.

Absolutely *all* the early pregnancy signs and symptoms to obsess about:

- Tingly or achy breasts
- Blue veins across chest and/or nipples
- Blue veins across tummy or thighs
- White creamy discharge
- Headaches
- Cramps
- Feeling thirsty
- Bloating
- Food aversions
- Food cravings
- Gas
- Diarrhoea
- Heartburn
- Exhaustion
- Enlarged nipples
- Darker nipples
- Heavy breasts
- Stuffy nose
- Nose bleeds
- Cramping above pubic bone
- Mood swings
- Dizziness or light-headedness
- Vivid dreams

Dreams of being pregnant
Watery cervical mucus
Lots of saliva in mouth
A 'pulling' sensation in uterus
A 'full' feeling in uterus
Twinges on left or right side of abdomen
Elevated (high) temperature
Lower back pain
Hunger
Bleeding gums
Depression
Sharp pains in uterus
Weepiness
Unusually warm skin
Taste of metal in mouth

'I don't even look at tampons or pads when I'm in the supermarket. I throw out any that might be in the bathroom cupboard during the TWW. I refuse to buy any until I actually have my period – that will jinx my luck.' **Jane, 31**

'I won't have an orgasm in the Two Week Wait because it might nudge the egg out or make the uterus shudder enough to un-stick it. Is that true?!' **Karen, 38**

Quick Quiz: Are you TWW bonkers yet?

1. Have you researched more on 'implantation bleeding' this week than any project you've ever had for work?

2. Have you checked your undies so many times in the office bathroom everyone thinks you must have a nasty urinary infection or an exotic tummy bug?
3. Have you read every single early pregnancy symptom ever recorded on www.twoweekwait.com?
4. Have you groped your boobs to see if they are tender so many times they are now tender?
5. Have you stared at your nipples so hard in the mirror checking for blue veins that now your whole chest area is a road map?
6. Have you thrust your breasts into your husband's face to ask if they are bigger so many times he no longer thinks you're being funny, you're just being weird?

If you answered 'yes' to most of the above then it's time to softly slap yourself and go anywhere where you won't be able to Google 'I feel crazy – could I be pregnant?' If you answered mostly 'no' to the above then you were too busy staring at your nipples to read the questions properly. Take test again.

> 'I never change our cat's kitty litter in the Two Week Wait – I make my husband do it. I also won't use chemical fertiliser in the garden, have sex or ride my bike to work.' **Emma, 34**

Keeping busy – Two Week Wait style

Here are some things to keep you busy during TWW:

- Take your temperature.
- Test your saliva for 'ferning'.
- Pray to God *this is the month!*
- Decide you'd better become religious.
- Grope your breasts to see if your nipples are sore.
- Promise to leave your breasts alone for at least an hour.
- Google 'I feel like sardines – am I pregnant???!!!'
- Refuse to stand near the washing machine or anything that vibrates.
- Take your temperature again.
- Refuse to use the photocopier at work.
- Stand in front of the mirror assessing the state of veins across your chest.
- Demand your husband tell you if your breasts look bigger, *any* bigger?
- Decide to stop being so 'berserk' and just go back to the computer and Google all your symptoms (again).

'I won't mow the lawn during the Two Week Wait or do anything with vibrations in it. I don't want to shake the embryo out. I want it to feel nice and safe.' **Karen, 38**

'I Google my symptoms so obsessively my husband has to carry me out of the house or take me away for the weekend. Anything so I'll get away from the computer for 10 minutes.' **Hannah, 31**

How to kill time in the TWW

Here are some ways to at least *try* to take your mind off things during the Two Week Wait:

- Concentrate on work (ooh that's right, work!).
- Go see a movie (no baby-themed flicks).
- Go into work on the weekend and clean up your desk.
- Send a thoughtful and personalised email to every friend you've been neglecting lately.
- Go for a long walk with a friend or relative who loves to chat.
- Clean out your wardrobe and give all your old clothes to charity.
- Feng shui your bedroom for better fertility (see 'Z is for zzzzz').
- Host a dinner party and spend a day slicing and dicing.

- Update your work wardrobe.
- Review your Bump & Grind Diary and make notes on what can be improved next cycle.
- Spend time with your partner just kissing and cuddling on the couch – no TTC talk!

> 'I used to wash my hair with baby shampoo during the TWW. It made my hair fuzzy and unmanageable but it was a TWW ritual I couldn't break. I also sniffed a lot of baby powder!' **Sam, 33**

> 'I have a shrine of good luck charms next to my bed. I have a tiny plastic baby doll, a dummy that a friend's baby dropped at our place (for good luck I think!) and a cake of baby soap. I used to sprinkle 'baby dust' around that I bought online too. I'm sure my partner thinks I'm a loser but he lets it slide.' **Kate, 28**

What's happening inside your body

- If sperm meets and penetrates the egg, it will fertilise the egg. Fertilisation takes about 24 hours.
- When fertilisation occurs, changes happen in the egg's surface to prevent other sperm from penetrating it. At the moment of fertilisation the genetic make-up becomes complete, including the sex of the baby.

- The egg begins to divide rapidly, growing into many cells. Three to four days after fertilisation in the fallopian tube, the egg enters the uterus.
- After entering the uterus, the egg attaches itself to the uterine lining or endometrium. This is called implantation. The cells are continually dividing.
- Human chorionic gonadotropin (HCG) will be present in the blood within a week of conception. It usually takes two to three weeks from conception for levels of HCG to be high enough to be detected in a home pregnancy test. The hormone is secreted by cells that eventually develop into the placenta.
- After implantation, some cells become the placenta while others become the embryo. About three weeks after ovulation the baby's brain, spinal cord, heart and other organs begin to form. The heart starts beating in week five.

With all this hopefully going on inside your body, you might want to avoid the following: drinking; smoking; taking recreational drugs; taking any prescription medication without clearing it with your GP; running a marathon.

'I don't ever say to someone to 'stop thinking about it' during the Two Week Wait. It's impossible not to be thinking about it! What is important is to help manage the anxiety of the waiting using herbs and acupuncture and whatever endeavours are calming to each individual woman, be that yoga or walking.' **Fertility acupuncturist and Chinese herbalist, Shauna Cason**

Implantation bleeding

Implantation bleeding usually takes place six to 12 days past ovulation and is variously described as spotting, a smear, a smudge or a little slick of blood in your undies. Once the egg becomes implanted in the uterus the 'burrowing in' might create a little bit of red, brown or pink spotting. If the spotting goes on longer than a day or two then it might be an early period. Only about 30 per cent of pregnant women experience implantation bleeding.

'I go to sleep every night with my hands on my belly talking to the embryo and wishing it luck. I try to make it feel warm and welcome in my body and then I say 'Now just f**king grab on!'' **Hannah, 31**

> 'I gave myself permission to stop falling apart in the Two Week Wait and just focused on work, my house and my relationship. When I thought about it, I just tried to stay busy. I cleaned every cupboard in our house!' **Lynne, 39**

Can anything help the embryo to implant in the Two Week Wait?

Chinese herbalists have their own special brews to keep the body warm after ovulation. 'Keeping your temperature up will help the production of progesterone,' says Chinese herbalist and acupuncturist Shauna Cason. She says a calm mind is also vital but don't worry if meditation sounds too much like hard work. If Googling all your symptoms at the computer calms you down and keeps you busy, then go for it.

Here's some more advice from Shauna:

It's very important to keep yourself warm during the Two Week Wait and to keep your basal body temperature (BBT) up. This indicates your progesterone levels are up which is what you want for a pregnancy.

Try to:

- *stay warm*
- *avoid cold drafts or going out in the rain or cold weather*
- *avoid eating raw foods*
- *avoid eating cold or frozen foods*

- *eat warming herbs and spices such as cinnamon and ginger*
- *eat warming foods – slow-cooked foods and stews are beneficial*
- *rest as much as you can*
- *keep a calm mind.*

Taking a pregnancy test

How soon can you take a pregnancy test? Most of us give it the official two weeks after sex at ovulation time, okay, nine days – okay, maybe eight days. It doesn't matter. Home pregnancy tests can be positive as early as 10 days after fertilisation – a couple of days before you miss your period. If you are going to test every morning from 10 days past ovulation though, you might want to buy some cheaper tests online well before the Two Week Wait kicks off. Remember, your first urine of the day is best and be warned: if you squint long enough at a test you will not only eventually see an extra blue line but purple spots (and then go cross-eyed).

> 'I take a test two mornings before I should get my period and on the actual day my period is due. It's become a ritual now and I feel like if I break it, I won't get pregnant.' **Karen, 38**

False negatives

So it's negative. It doesn't mean you're not pregnant. It might mean the HCG hasn't shown up in your urine yet. Take another test tomorrow morning. If it's still negative at the end of the Two Week Wait but you feel pregnant, see your GP for a blood test to confirm. I have a couple of TTC friends who didn't get a positive test until they were a week past the Two Week Wait and only a blood test confirmed they were pregnant. They just *felt* different. Remember, a woman's intuition is a powerful insight into what's going on in her body.

Have a plan

Having a plan about what you're going to do if the pregnancy test is positive *and* if it's negative might be a way of keeping you calm this month.

Positive plan

- How are you going to tell your partner?
- Who are you going to tell first?
- Do you have your supplements in order? Folic acid is the one you'll need to start immediately if you are not already taking it – at least 400mcg a day.
- What are you going to post in your favourite TTC forum online?
- How are you going to celebrate?

Negative plan

- When will you take another test?
- Will you wait a day or two?

- What's your period party this month? Plan a bloody good one!
- Will you jump into another cycle or give it a few months and rethink?
- What might you do differently the next cycle – try acupuncture, overhaul your lifestyle, go see a naturopath for more comprehensive supplements?
- Who is a good shoulder to cry on for a few days – if you need to?
- Will you see how hubby is coping too and take him out for a beer?
- Will you congratulate yourself on getting through the TWW? You should – you're amazing!

'Get plenty of sleep and stay calm. Avoid as much stress as possible. If trying to meditate is more than you can cope with and the idea of sitting down and crossing your legs is stressful just do something rhythmical like walking or even dancing. Anything that will give you a calm mind is vital in the Two Week Wait.' **Fertility acupuncturist and Chinese herbalist, Shauna Cason**

TWW affirmations

'Healthy eggs meet healthy sperm – now set up camp!'

'I am calm and rested.'

'I am warm and comfortable.'
'Healthy body, happy heart.'
'I am not a nutcase (at least, not completely!).'
'Everything is going to be okay – no matter what.'
'There's always next month.'
'Every cycle gets me closer and closer.'
'I'll keep up my healthy living because my
skinny jeans are starting to look smokin'!'

PS: The essence of the Two Week Wait is that when it comes to signs and symptoms, nothing means anything and everything means something. That means you're allowed to be crazy for two weeks - at least!

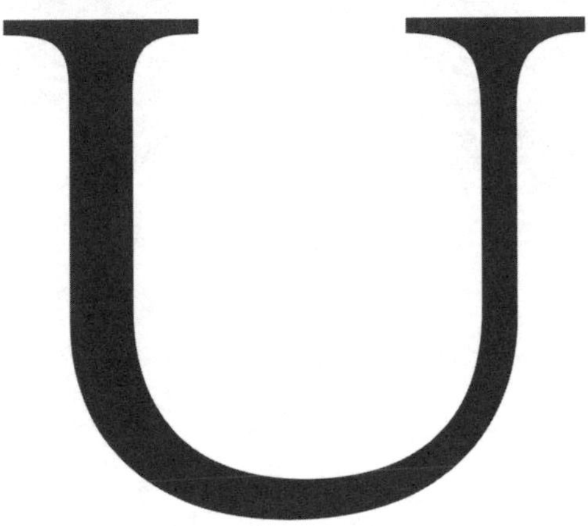

U is for us against the world

When you're TTC it can sometimes feel as if you're living on a little island in the Sea of Fertility. It's just you and your hubby on your little island, battling isolation and difference while secretly hoping no-one from the Sea of Fertility swims by for a cup of coconut juice or, worse, brings any of their

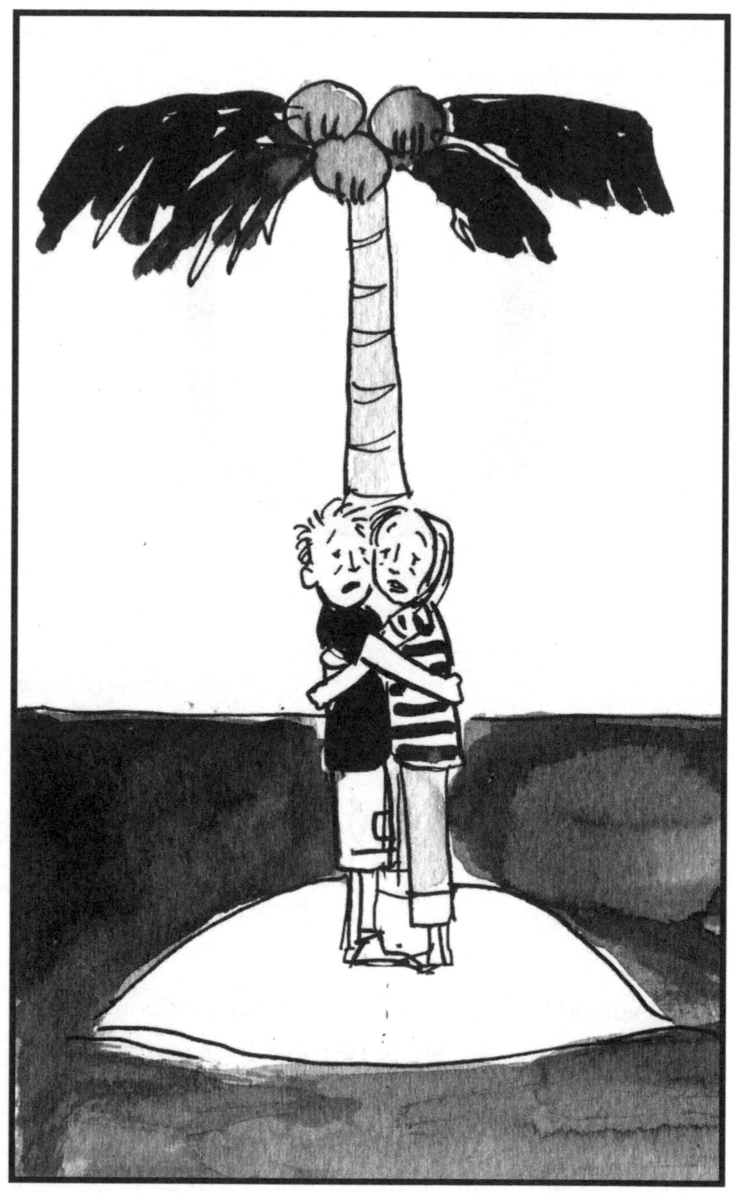

little tribe with them. It can be lonely. But it's often so hard sailing away from the island when you don't feel like paddling or, worse, you almost sank last time.

When we were about a year into TTC and I was just starting to get a *tad* cranky about it, I went to a barbecue to find a Smug Fertility Goddess at the grill turning the tofu. She assured me she wasn't even *trying* to get pregnant, and she wasn't sure if having a baby was the right 'move' for them. And then she smiled smugly into her ginger beer.

It didn't seem fair.

I spent the entire car ride home crying – why does this keep happening! It's *not* fair! And I felt sad for my husband Ben. Would this ever happen for him? I just wanted to hide away from the world with Ben until I felt better about mixing with The Fertiles (or got pregnant).

I found lots of ways to avoid pregnant friends and friends with babies for a while but I'm not sure if hiding away from the world was very good for us. It's often too much pressure on you both. For a while there I didn't want Ben to talk about our fertility issues and his friends simply had to guess why he wasn't drinking beer, or at times even coffee. It kept things semi-private for me on my island but it added to the pressure on him. He wasn't ashamed or embarrassed about it, so why did it matter if people knew we were trying? There might be something in letting a few outsiders dock their canoe on your shore – especially if they bring a fresh perspective and encouragement. It's also great finding people who offer all of this but have been through the TTC experience and understand your need for privacy too. It's only when you let a few outsiders dock at your island that you realise how far-reaching and how complicated trying for a baby actually is. It can feel like an island (and you can make it one, like I did) but the truth is, there are thousands, no, millions of couples going through this too. That doesn't make your experience feel any less lonely at times, but it's good to know you're not alone. And if you don't want to feel lonely, you don't have to.

'I knew I was leaning too much on my partner after I screamed at him that he didn't understand. Of course he didn't understand. How could he know what TTC felt like for me? He's a guy! I soon found some women in the same boat online to talk to.' **Holly, 32**

Quick Quiz: Are you too 'us against the world'?

1. Have you stopped planning social events because they'll interfere with you and your partner's healthy living or weight loss efforts for TTC?
2. Have you stopped going to social events because you can't face pregnant women or women with babies without your partner by your side?
3. Does your partner know way too much about your cycle?

4. When people invite you both away for a weekend, is your cycle the first thing you think about?
5. Have you forgotten the last time you simply hung out with friends and were genuinely interested in *their* problems?
6. Have you forgotten the last time you did something fun as a couple that had nothing to do with TTC?

If you answered 'yes' to most of the above then you've been living on your island so long your hair has officially gone from 'windswept' to 'sea wench' (don't worry, it's still a cute look). If you answered 'no' to most of the above then you've been keeping your big toe in the water and that might be a good thing.

Hiding out

It's so easy to dump all your fears and anxieties on your partner when you're TTC. You trust him, he wants this too and he's the person closest to you. So you can't help but leave out most of the censoring you do at work or when you're with friends and family. Your partner gets the unscripted, unedited version of you and let's face it, she can be a bit nutty and negative. While it's great that TTC will bring you closer, you don't want to be so close that you suffocate each other and make it even harder. Don't dump every little detail on him, don't expect him to understand how you're feeling every day, don't use him as a punching bag when you're angry and disappointed.

Psychologist and IVF counsellor Lynne Quayle says we should look at our relationship like a tall building, always being mindful of repairing cracks and making sure the foundations stay nice and sturdy. That might mean finding another avenue to let your unedited self out for a run. A counsellor, your confidante or your diary can cop it. Diaries are great listeners. Venting all your feelings and fears on paper is a great release when you're TTC. Start the Bump & Grind Diary (see page 136) and get scribbling. I promise it won't mind how grumpy you sound.

> 'Self-awareness and relationship awareness are critical here. IVF (or other) couples are usually pretty resilient individuals but sometimes, despite how critical or urgent each and every cycle seems to be, it can be in the best interest of the individuals and the relationship to take time out to reduce the degree of stress, check the foundations, patch the cracks and plan how to avoid overstress in the future.'
>
> **Psychologist and IVF counsellor, Lynne Quayle**

Mixing with The Fertiles

A baby won't complete a couple. The same problems will still be there – and then some. A baby adds to the pressure on a relationship rather than taking it away. You don't have to watch a couple for long to see just how much extra pressure a baby puts on them. When you're TTC it's sometimes hard to see the realities of having a child, you just *want* one. But it is good to keep some perspective and sometimes it's nice to walk away from a date with The Fertiles feeling content that it's just you and your partner (for now!).

> 'I like to remind myself that other couples have other problems like infidelity or the guy doesn't like being a father – or whatever. I imagine them fighting all the time. It makes me feel better!!'
>
> **Lou, 40**

Party people

Friends with babies (unless they battled the Baby Gods) rarely worry about healthy lifestyle issues when it comes to fertility. They may have just sprogged up after a boozy night ('I didn't even know I was ovulating!'). So when it comes to mixing with them, it's important to keep in mind they have no idea that you don't drink as much as you used to, don't eat crappy food and probably won't want to stay out until 4 a.m. If you don't want them to know you're TTC then you just have to blur the truth a little here and there. Here are some excuses for why you're not playing up:

'I'm detoxing.'

'It's a dare I have with some work friends – no drinking for a month.'

'I'm on a health kick – no booze or coffee for six weeks.'

'I'm driving.'

'I have a headache.'

'I'm not feeling well, I might go home early; but let's catch up during the week.'

> 'Friends who don't know we're TTC think I'm just a mad health nut. I think I annoy them.' **Kim, 37**

Some of The Fertiles will give you a hard time for leaving an event (or not going), some won't mind at all and some will guess that you are trying to knock yourself up rather than knock yourself out on a Saturday night. You can't worry too much about what other people think. Say no to things you just know will involve compulsory drinking and don't feel bad. Reschedule catch-ups with them for breakfast and go out for fresh juices and eggs rather than beers and cigarettes.

How to leave the island

- Plan a few social events.
- Turn *up* to a few social events.
- Make contact with your old friends – not your 'couple' friends.
- Do things without your partner on weekends.

PS: You don't need to leave your island on a jet ski; go slow, make him row.

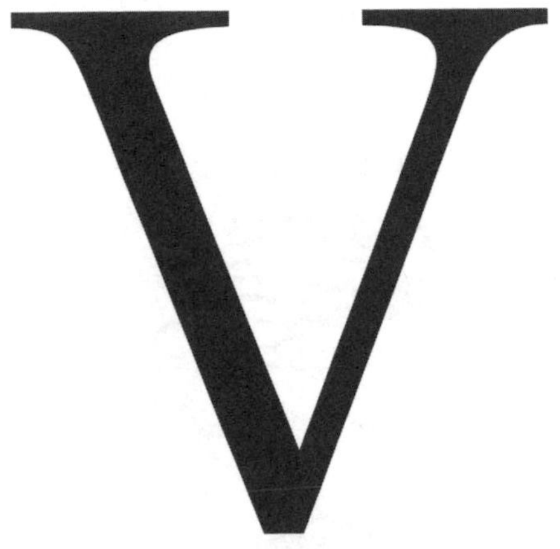

V is for visualisations and magical stuff

I used to be a bit of a girl scout about TTC. When we were first told our unexplained infertility might be due to *emotional* reasons I stuck that in my gingham rucksack. That sounded too faffy and silly for this sensible girl so I diligently went back to following the 'rules': calculating my dates and

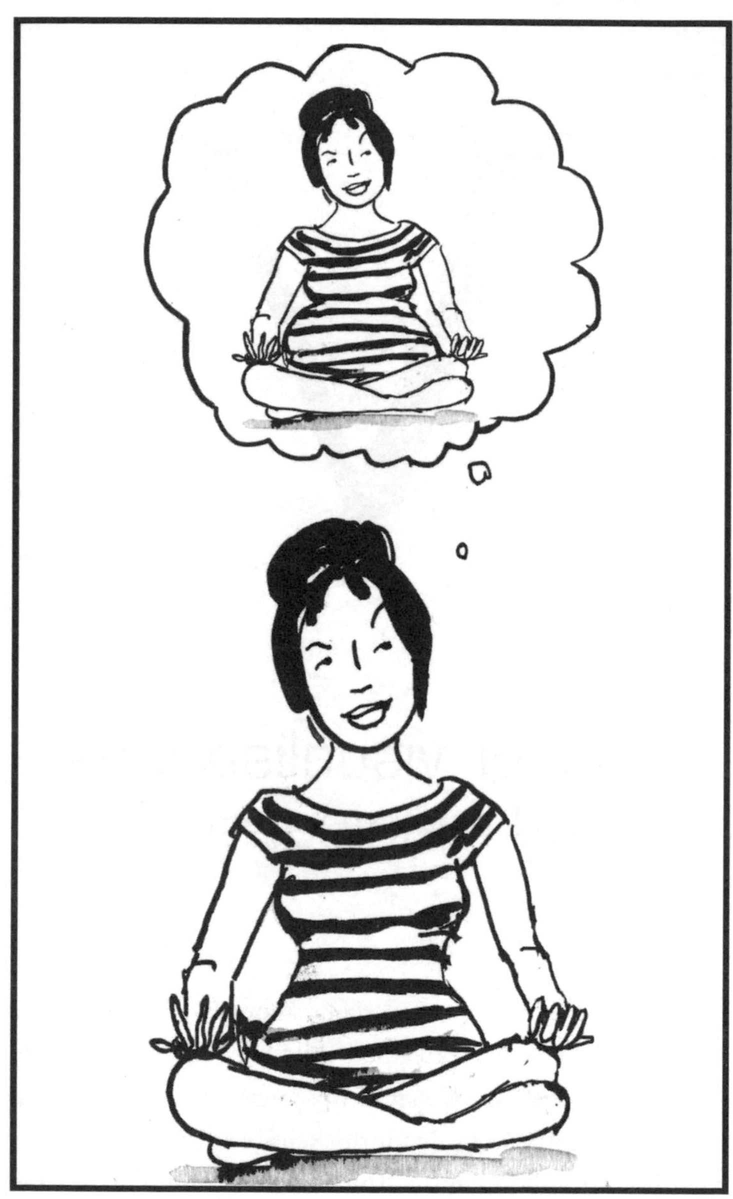

a militant sex schedule, while secretly quashing all my fears and anxieties beneath my left fallopian tube. It took me 18 months to acknowledge that the 'rules' weren't working and that bracing myself for failure, over-analysing and being so-called sensible might be *preventing* a pregnancy.

And so I opened my gingham rucksack and tried acupuncture and reflexology. I even tried visualisations, meditation and all that magical stuff we sensible girl scouts don't tend to sing songs about. But we should. The truth is, so often, they *work*.

Here's a little of what happened to me when I started trying to find myself – or at least get a glimpse of her …

Visualisation and self-talk

One of the first things the Fertility Sisters instructed me to do was to visualise myself as a mum, really see myself in the situation. What did I look like? What did Ben look like as a dad? At the time I burst into tears and sobbed 'I've never really imagined that before!' to which one of them clicked her tongue and raised her eyebrow as much to say 'Oh dear, she's one stressed-out little nut, that's for sure!'

In order to turn myself into Mother Earth – or at least knock myself up – I desperately needed to *believe* I could get pregnant. I needed to see it clearly. So it took some foraging around in my head *and* my heart for answers. I found some interesting stuff in there. I somehow believed that I might not deserve a baby. Did I really deserve a baby when I already had such a great relationship and a good job? Who said I could have all that? I couldn't, could I? I was unconsciously bracing myself for not getting what I wanted. I didn't realise at the time that bracing myself was part of the problem. The Fertility Sisters said this was a message to my body *not* to let it happen. I had to let go of all that and realise that it *could* happen for me. I could have what I wanted. And even if it didn't happen straight away, I knew that I deserved it to, eventually. Phew!

Retrain the brain

This is what used to run through my head when we were TTC: *I can't get pregnant. It's not fair. I must be infertile. It's never going to happen.*

And you know what? My body delivered on all those messages. I couldn't get pregnant. It wasn't fair. We had unexplained infertility. It didn't happen for 18 months.

What we tell ourselves is who we become. So what do you tell yourself each day? It's never going to happen? It's all up to me? I must be infertile? I'm running out of time? Oh God, what if this doesn't happen soon? It's not fair?

Shut up head, already!

It might be time to listen to that little voice in your head (no, the other one!) and if she's a negative grumpy-bum like mine used to be about TTC then it might be time to start shutting her down. With some practice I could hear her worst-case scenario popping into my mind ('It's never going to happen') and I'd flick it out of there and replace it with the best possible outcome ('It's going to happen soon!').

Just for today, observe those negative thoughts resting in your mind, flick them out of there and replace them (say it out loud if you have to) with the best possible outcome. For example: 'This is never going to happen for us.'

Replace with: 'This is going to happen for us exactly when it's meant to – and soon!'

Or: 'I can't stand TTC any more; it's so frustrating.'

Replace with: 'TTC is making us stronger than ever.'

I reckon you'll be happier and more hopeful. And I know, I know, hope isn't going to unblock a fallopian tube or boost a sperm count, no. But the way you see the world comes from within you. So the way you see TTC comes from within you, right? You can go bracing yourself for the worst-case scenario like I did or you can jump back into it expecting the best. You deserve the best possible outcome. And you're going to get it too.

Affirmations when you're TTC

If you feel that negative voice starting to take over, try saying some of these positive affirmations to yourself:

'My body is prime-time ready for a baby.'

'*Now* is the perfect time for a baby.'

'I've never been more ready.'

'We deserve to be a happy little family.'
'I am going to *kick arse* as a mum.'
'Healthy eggs, healthy sperm.'
'I am a healthy and hot yummy-mummy-in-the-making.'
'I love the fertility super foods pumpkin seeds and sardines.' (Hmm, maybe leave that one out.)

Meditation

It's too easy to think about what might *not* happen to us, isn't it? Those who believe in the connection between meditation and improving fertility say we should start focusing on what we *want* to happen to us instead. That means whatever you focus on with true understanding and conviction is what you will draw into your life. The key to meditation and improving your fertility is to see what you want, see the outcome and *live* in the result as if it is already happening. That doesn't mean living in a fantasy world – hey, we still have to turn up to work on time. It means embracing your desire (having a baby), visualising it (seeing that baby) and allowing yourself to feel all the happiness this brings. It's about practising in your mind what is possible.

Want to try? Here's a sample meditation a super-spiritual friend of mine helped me devise for you.

Fertility-booster meditation

Find a safe, quiet and comfortable spot to rest (you can lie down or sit up, whatever is comfy), then close your eyes. Become aware of your breathing; rhythmically breathe in and out, in and out, without forcing your breath. Let go of any thoughts that may come up, don't get caught on any, just see them and let them go. Now imagine a white light slowly filling your body from head to toe, healing and soothing you inside and out. Feel the energy in your lower body and imagine creating a space for new life to come into you. Imagine that space as emerald green (emerald green is the aura associated with fertility).

While keeping that green light in your belly, bring orange (for health and energy) to the rest of your body. Allow yourself to smile, and keep breathing. Silently talk to your baby-to-be that's coming – whatever pops into your mind (don't worry if it makes you laugh). Allow yourself to be happy.

Take a few deeper breaths. Bring a feeling of complete joy to yourself and allow it to wash over you. Then slowly open your eyes and become aware of your surroundings.

There are lots of ways to meditate and the only rule is that you give yourself the time to try. It can take a while to master being still and having a quiet mind but even just stopping and creating some quiet down time will make you feel more at peace. Remember, when we are rela– sorry, chilled out, the body is free to do its work – like regulate hormones and produce healthy eggs.

> 'Meditation for me is just about lying in my bed before I go to sleep and talking to my body; well, my ovaries.' **Lynne, 39**

Reflexology

Kick off your Jimmy Choos! Reflexology is fast gaining a reputation as a fertility super-tool. The traditional healing art dates back to the ancient Egyptians and Chinese, and involves manipulation of pressure points in the feet. Practitioners claim the soles of the feet are like little maps of the inside of your body and are linked to bodily systems including the fallopian tubes and ovaries. By massaging different points, energy pathways can be unblocked to help the body regain natural balance and heal itself. Some points in the foot are linked to a woman's egg production and by manipulating the area through massage imbalances which hamper pregnancy can be corrected. The best part about reflexology is that once you get handy at it, you can practise it at home. Find out where the special spots are for increasing energy flow to the ovaries and uterus and instruct your partner – your new masseuse – where to go. My hubby Ben and I did lots of reflexology (about half an hour every night) in the month we conceived. I wanted to keep it up throughout the entire pregnancy but he got sick of me shoving my feet in his lap every night. So unfair!

Does it work?

It worked for us. It might work for you too. And no matter what, a good foot rub is only going to help you chill out and spend more quality time with your partner. Fertility-friendly oils to use for massage include lavender and rose or, less fancy, good old olive oil from your pantry will do the job.

Should you rub *his* feet? Well yes, that will help too but let him get good at massaging your feet first! It should take an hour session *every* night for at *least* three weeks …

Acupuncture

Acupuncture, often combined with Chinese herbs, has been used for centuries to treat infertility. An acupuncturist inserts tiny needles into various points on the body which reside on channels or meridians to stimulate energy flow or *chi*. Acupuncture won't fix tubal adhesions as a result of pelvic inflammatory disease or endometriosis, but you can still benefit because of improved ovarian and follicular function. It's been shown that acupuncture increases blood flow to the endometrium helping to create a rich, thick lining. It's often combined with Chinese herbs to treat elevated follicle stimulating hormone (FSH), repeated pregnancy loss, unexplained infertility, luteal phase defects, hyperprolactinemia, polycystic ovarian syndrome (PCOS) with anovulatory cycles, and male factors including men affected with sperm-DNA-fragmentation. That's a lot of healing for such tiny needles!

'Acupuncture facilitates follicular development, regulates hormones and calms the mind. It can support progesterone levels, supply blood to the endometrium, and ameliorate the possible side effects of IVF drugs. Overall, what Chinese medicine does is encourage the body to self-regulate.' **Fertility acupuncturist and Chinese herbalist, Shauna Cason**

What happens?

Forget about images you might have of your tummy or pelvic area covered in needles on your first visit. Needles are most likely going to be inserted in your toes, lower legs and wrists. You will lie on your back fully clothed (kick your shoes and socks off and roll up your trousers) on a comfy table while the acupuncturist gently 'screws' the tiny needles into your skin. It doesn't hurt but it does feel strange.

Once the needles are in, you lie on the table resting for about half an hour. The lights will be low, there might be some soft music playing and no doubt some yummy oils will be burning nearby. Many women find the practice so relaxing they'll nod off for the entire treatment. I found my legs felt heavy and achy the first visit (very normal, apparently) and I got lots of exciting and strong visualisations of babies and children on the second visit (visualisations are common too). While the needles had me more stressed out than blissed out I could definitely feel them *doing* something. After half an hour or so the acupuncturist will then come in and take the needles out. Your legs and wrists will feel completely normal. And no, there won't be any blood.

'If a woman is going to look into herbs and acupuncture combined, the length of treatment time will depend on the woman's age and the reason for infertility. In a relatively young, healthy woman where there are no obvious impediments to conception Chinese medicine is a very good option to explore. In these cases it's just often a matter of regulating the hormones and this may be dealt with relatively quickly – three to six months. The beauty of Chinese medicine is that it aims to heal without the trauma and detrimental side effects often experienced when using fertility drugs. Having said that, I believe there are many cases that will still require IVF and Chinese medicine can be employed alongside and with great effect during each phase of an IVF process.'

Fertility acupuncturist and Chinese herbalist, Shauna Cason

Some advice

- See a traditional fertility specialist first to see what your fertility issues are (if any), as acupuncture will not help problems needing surgical intervention such as a blocked fallopian tube.

- Make sure your acupuncturist is trained and licensed and has lots of experience.
- Consider getting a referral from your fertility specialist to a reputable acupuncturist specialising in fertility management.
- Or, book in with an acupuncturist who your friends have enjoyed success with. The best acupuncturists are often found via word of mouth.
- Give yourself plenty of time to get to appointments and then get back into your day – rushing in and out of a session defeats the purpose of 'relaxation'.

Chinese herbs

Chinese herbs have a long history in aiding fertility. The herbal treatment of infertility and miscarriage reportedly dates back to 200 AD. No one special herb is considered useful for improving fertility but rather, more than 150 different herbs are dished out in complex formulas each containing 15 or more ingredients. Each formula is created with the individual's needs in mind to correct a functional or organic problem. The most prominent ingredients are derived from roots, barks, leaves, flowers and fruits.

Herbs are ingested via tablets, granules or decoctions (teas). Some of the treatment plans involve using a single herbal combination regularly, while other situations require using two, or even three, different formulas at different times of the menstrual cycle. How do you know the herbs are working? You'll have more energy, sleep better and feel better physically overall. Of course the ultimate sign of successful treatment is that you'll get pregnant!

Chinese herbs are most commonly combined with acupuncture in treating infertility. If you are undergoing IVF or about to embark on IVF, talk to your fertility specialist if you are considering taking any Chinese herbs.

PS: If to you 'meditating' is just time spent thinking about what you need to do tomorrow, just take some time out for things that make you happy. Singing in the car, a long bath, knitting, watching reality TV. Whatever switches you off will help turn baby-making on.

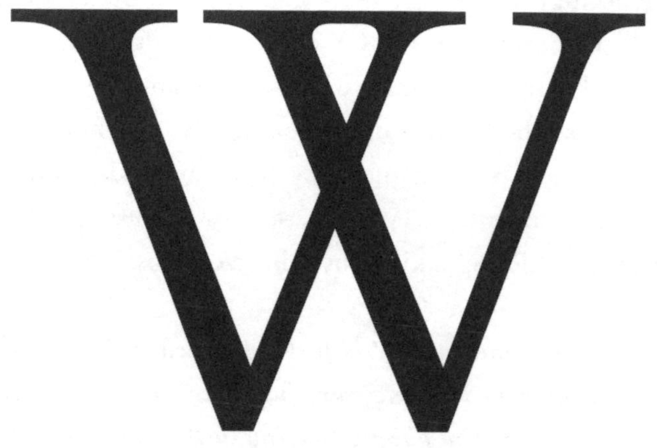

W is for Way of the Bunny Rabbit

I know what you're thinking: this is going to be stoopid, right? Bunny rabbits? Alas, when you're battling the Baby Gods and nothing is working, it's sometimes nice to 'walk to a different tune' or in this case, hop to one. In other words, try something different this cycle. The Way of The Bunny Rabbit

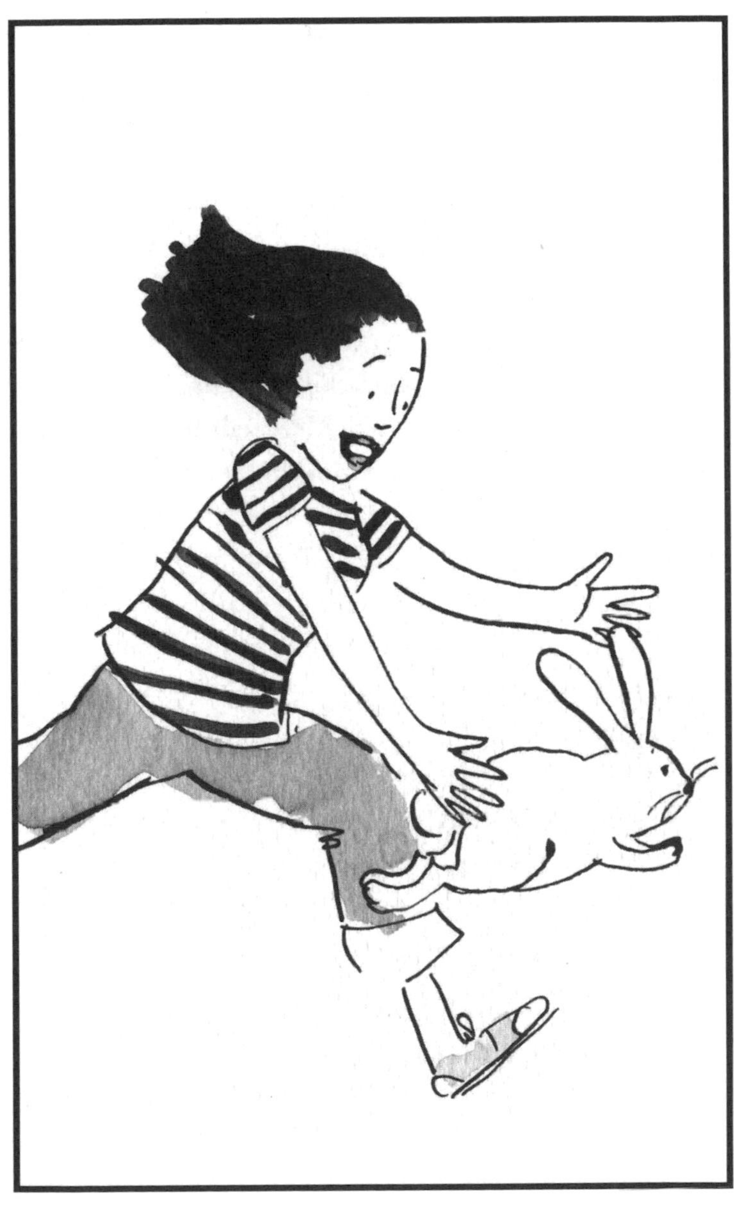

made a healthy pregnancy possible for Ben and I in just three weeks (or one cycle) after 18 miserable months of TTC. Was it a fluke? I don't think so. From the moment I started taking better care of my health and, more importantly, my *heart*, I felt different – lighter, happier, freer, more *fertile*. Remember my very first visit to the Fertility Sisters? They had said that if I was a bunny rabbit the message I was sending my body was that there wasn't enough green grass around to feed little bunnies. I was too stressed and lacking in basic nutrients in my diet for good reproductive health, they said, and when I dealt with my head-stress, my body would follow.

Amid all the good living (and loving!) an image kept popping into my head. It was a bunny rabbit. I want to include all this funny bunny business because it just might work for you too. And fast. The Way of the Bunny Rabbit has six basic principles:

1. An alkaline diet
2. The right supplements
3. No thinking, excessive charting or worrying
4. Lots of meditation, positive self-talk and smiling
5. Getting your goop on
6. Sex, like *bunny rabbits*

1. An alkaline diet

An alkaline diet is one that is made up of 80 per cent alkaline foods and 20 per cent acidic foods. Of course, there are neutral foods in between. It's important not to get too stressed about your diet and doing it all perfectly (because that's too hard!) but your body – especially your cervical mucus – will thank you if you load up on alkaline foods and stay away from acidic foods and drinks where you can when you're TTC.

Alkaline foods and drinks include: lemons, watermelon, dried dates and figs, kelp, limes, mango, melons, papaya, parsley, seedless grapes, watercress, seaweed, asparagus, kiwifruit, passionfruit, pears, pineapple, raisins, umeboshi plums (Japanese pickled plums), vegetable juices, apples, apricots, avocados, bananas, berries, carrots, garlic, peaches, pumpkin, lettuce.

Acidic foods and drinks to avoid include: beer, brown sugar, chicken, chocolate, coffee, jams, jellies, white pasta, black tea, white rice, beef, carbonated soft drinks, lamb, pastries and cakes, pork, white sugar.

Neutral foods to be enjoyed moderately include: butter, cream, milk, oils, yoghurt, blueberries, brazil nuts, cheeses, dried beans, egg whites, olives, pecans, plums, prunes, bran, cashews, cereals, lentils, popcorn, rye bread, walnuts.

See 'H is for healthy living' for a TTC eating plan but go big on alkaline foods where you can. I felt a whole lot cleaner on an alkaline diet and slept much better too. It was like I was giving my body a break to do its proper work – to make quality eggs (hold the hollandaise).

2. The right supplements

A one-stop preconception supplement will work for lots of women but for others, like me, a little more help is needed.

The best way to go about getting the right supplements for both you and your partner is to visit a really good naturopath, preferably one who specialises in fertility management. You may have a pretty good diet, already joined the chai latte set and given up grog (and realised you do need alcohol to have a good time at parties!) but you still might need help. Here's why:

- Smoking, drinking, tea, coffee and cola drinks draw heavily on your zinc supplies (and we know zinc is the TTC champion).
- Stress increases the need for zinc and all the B-complex vitamins.
- The pill may have adversely affected your folate levels.
- Soils used to grow vegetables may be depleted of vital essential nutrients.
- Your body needs extra essential nutrients to detoxify it of pollutants such as heavy metals.

PS: My naturopath said the silver fillings in my teeth were giving me a high reading of mercury (which was adding to failing fertility) so I had them whipped out by a dentist and replaced with safe ceramic fillings. The cost was not something to smile about.

Supplements – where to start?

So you have an appointment with your new best friend – your fertility-friendly naturopath – and you have no idea what supplements you might need or what to ask about. Here's a basic guide that might help you raise some talking points …

Zinc is the fertility champ. If you have a deficiency in zinc, it can upset the menstrual cycle and slow down the metabolism of protein – necessary for the production of eggs. In men, a deficiency in zinc lowers sperm count and levels of testosterone, and can cause poor sperm motility.

Vitamin B6 is essential for the production and balance of female sex hormones. In his book *Fit For Fertility*, Dr Michael Dooley says 'Research has shown that women who had previously had difficulty in conceiving saw a marked increase in their fertility after being given B6. Periods were regulated and the incidence of pregnancy rose.' Ask about that!

Folic acid has been proven to help prevent babies developing neural tube defects. It is generally recommended women start taking 400mcg of folic acid for three months before trying to conceive until at least 12 weeks into pregnancy. The pill can deplete your folate levels.

Vitamin C is a powerful antioxidant that can improve sperm motility and quantity.

Vitamin E is another powerful antioxidant. Also in his book *Fit For Fertility*, Dr Michael Dooley says: 'There is evidence to suggest that taking antioxidants like C and E can significantly reduce age-related ovulation decline; clearly such findings could have an enormous impact on older women's fertility.' I'll say! Ask your naturopath for more info!

Iron is said to be a good guard against miscarriage. We need iron for the formation of red blood cells, to carry oxygen to organs and muscles and for healthy bones. It is best absorbed when taken with vitamin C (a glass of orange juice is fine) particularly for non-haem (from non-animal/non-meat) iron as very little iron from non-haem sources is absorbed unless ingested with vitamin C.

Some questions to ask your naturopath

- Does taking vitamins B6 and C aid the absorption of zinc?
- What's all the fuss about soy products around ovulation? Can I still drink soy milk?
- If vitamin A is something to be avoided in large amounts in pregnancy, why are we told to take it when trying to conceive?
- How can you test us both for zinc levels?
- Should I go see my dentist and have my silver fillings taken out? Will you test my urine for heavy metals?

3. No thinking, excessive charting or worrying

Permission to stop thinking? What do you think of that?! Well, maybe keep thinking (a little) but not so much mental gymnastics regarding TTC that you could put the Russians to shame. In other words, when you find yourself Googling yet again for infertility or why we 30-somethings are supposedly 'reproductively challenged', then just stop. Close that link and walk away. Too much information just isn't good for you. I used to chow down so much information on fertility that I'm sure it made me infertile. I just couldn't stop thinking about what I was doing wrong and where all the TTC was going …

It was a relief to stop all the researching and planning and try to simply trust that my body would do what nature intended it to do. I once went to see a psychic to see when I'd get pregnant (uh huh) and he said 'Don't take the A to B route to get what you want, go with the flow'. I wanted to shove the £45 I paid to hear 'go with the flow' in his peace pipe. But he was right. Taking the A to B route just made me anxious, hard on myself and stressed that I wasn't getting there quick enough. When I relinquished control to the Baby Gods and let go enough to go with the flow (man), it happened, I got pregnant.

When it comes to charting, it was also a relief to stop *recording* everything and just listen to my body a little closer. I still used an OPK the month we conceived but I'd abandoned any kind of sex schedule – we just did it every night for a week with a few mornings thrown in.

Quitting worrying was the hardest. I'm not sure who I'd be without a little worry here and there. But when it came to TTC I eventually realised I had worried so much in 18 months I just couldn't worry about it a day longer.

I gave up control, handed it back to the Baby Gods and *stopped worrying.* There is so much to worry about when you're TTC. Did we time that right? Did I stand on my head long enough? Was the sperm good enough? Will it implant? Will it stick? Will I survive the Two Week Wait? Will I – arrrghhh! Worrying doesn't actually *do* anything. It doesn't change anything or keep you in control. It just adds to the stress of TTC, which works against you. It's not easy but keep a watch on your worrying and cut back, cut down, and stop.

What are you worried about? Write it down here:

....

....

....

Uh huh, keep going …

....

....

....

What else?

....

....

....

So what can be done about the above? How much of it is just plain dumb old worry? Try to write solutions for the things you can change and ignore the things you can't. Perhaps write these things down in the back of your Bump & Grind Diary, along with the solutions you've come up with.

> 'Unfortunately, unlike improving our golf stroke or essay writing skills, it doesn't seem that we can get better at falling pregnant by concentrating harder or exclusively on the topic.'
>
> **Psychologist and IVF counsellor, Lynne Quayle**

4. Lots of meditation, positive self-talk and smiling

Meditation and *smiling*? I can hear a grumble among the busy career types. I don't have time! When it comes to TTC, it might be time to make time. It's time to stop being so busy. It's time to tell yourself that everything is going to be okay, and to try to be happy. What we tell ourselves is who we are. And we know the health benefits in taking the time to unwind and be a little more balanced in our lives. No more excuses. Take a little more time out each day to meditate, or just sit still and be pampered. And *smile*. You're a bunny rabbit, there's nothing to worry about, it's the perfect time to have a baby, there's plenty of green grass. Everything is going to be okay. ☺

5. Getting your goop on

On my very first visit to the Fertility Sisters they asked me three things. One, are you as strrrressed out as you seem? Two, is your husband as preoccupied with this as you are? And three, do you get plenty of cervical mucus around ovulation each month? I answered yes, sometimes and I'm not really sure.

'Not sure about cervical mucus,' they clicked their tongues, eyeing each other like worried aunts. 'You need plenty of goop, it's almost impossible to get pregnant naturally without a lot of goop helping things along.'

Goop? You know, that *stuff.*

Here I'd been worrying about Ben's gizz and nagging it into better shape, but I didn't realise cervical mucus was just as crucial. Good goop helps the sperm get to the egg. While she's out there on her 24-hour mission to get hit on, the sperm is looking for an easy entrance into the club. Healthy, slippery goop helps him slide by the bouncers and straight to your egg at the bar. He could live for 72 hours in there (imagine his hangover!).

A-grade natural goop:

- permits a passage of sperm through the cervix and uterus
- provides nutritional support and protection for sperm
- neutralises acidity in the vagina during a woman's fertile time
- helps prevent infections
- shields the sperm and sustains sperm movement.

See 'K is for keeping track' for way too much information on what your goop should look like at different stages of your cycle.

How do I improve my goop?

An alkaline diet, reducing stress, drinking lots of water and getting regular exercise will all help you get your goop on.

Is there any fake goop I can use instead?

If you still need a little help getting things moving along, there are some very good sperm-friendly personal lubricants out there. We used PreSeed for the first time the month we got pregnant. You can buy PreSeed online. It's a clear, slippery liquid that you squirt *up there* a little while before sex (to let it 'warm up').

6. Sex, like *bunny rabbits*

Here's where the bunny bit kicks in, sorry, hops to it. This month, maybe abandon your every-other-day sex schedule and just do it as soon as you see that line in your OPK, then again that night, the next morning and the day after that too. Make it fun – and fast. With all the researching, the charting, the worrying and the planning in TTC, we can sometimes forget that making a baby comes down to this very simple act. Egg, meet sperm.

Just have fun sex. A lot. Hop to it!

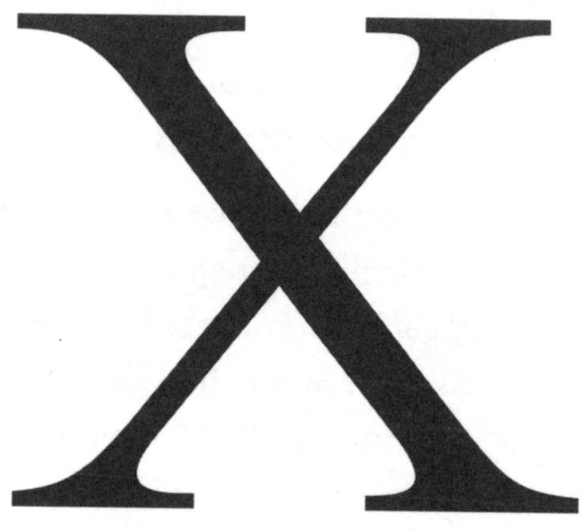

X is for kisses and cuddles

Somewhere between Ready, Set, Sex! and 'Why isn't this working?' you realise your relationship is going to be tested. And then tested some more. TTC can sometimes take the fun out of your relationship, or even drain the love out. It's important to get out of the TTC grind every now and then and just kiss and cuddle, make each other laugh and do

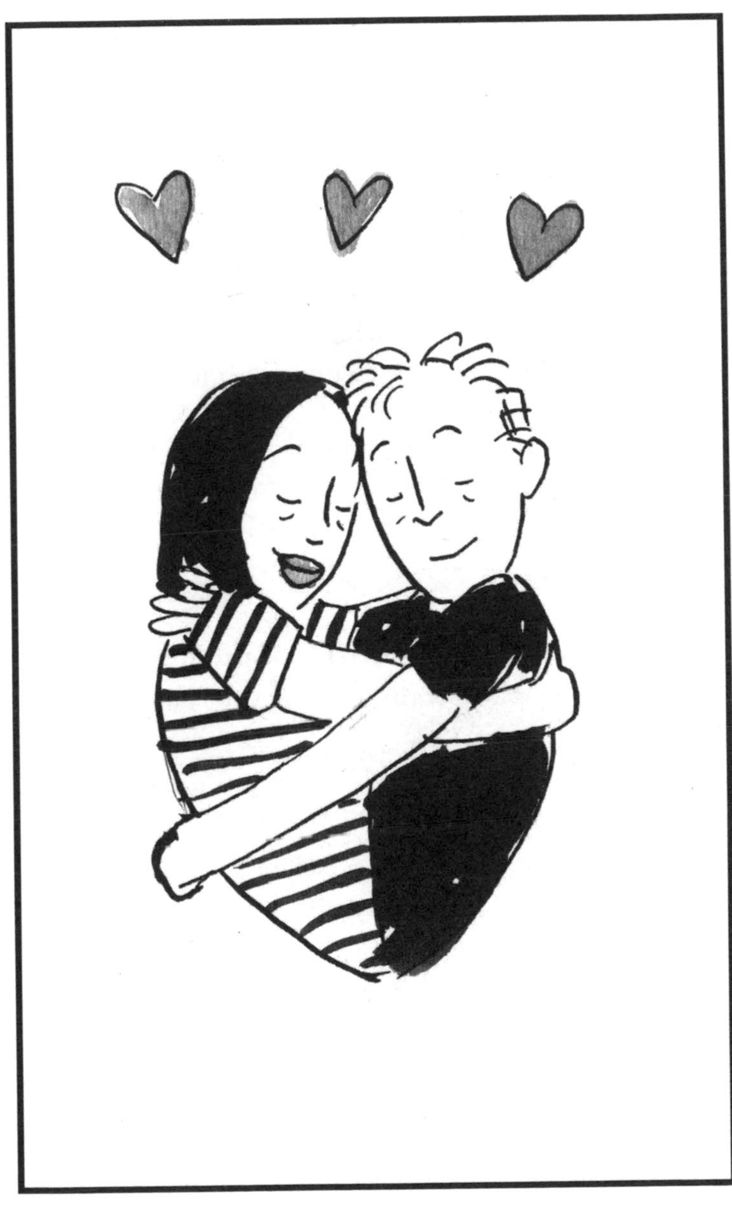

things together that don't involve sperm-friendly lubricants. *Your relationship is the most important part of baby-making.* It really is. You'll need plenty of love around for you, your partner and the baby you're going to make this month.

> 'I absolutely tested our relationship when we first started TTC. We argued all the time about lifestyle problems and who was to blame or who was doing all the work to make a baby possible. But when I thought about it my relationship really was the steadying force when everything else felt out of control. And I woke up to that eventually!' **Kim, 37**

Quick Quiz: Have I let TTC drain out the love?

1. Can you remember the last time you laughed out loud?
2. Can you remember the last time you had sex just for fun?
3. Have you stopped getting excited about silly stuff?
4. Have you had any quality time to yourself when you weren't worrying about TTC for months?
5. Have you made an effort to spend time with friends lately?
6. Can you plan your life beyond this cycle?

If you answered mostly 'no' to the above then you might have let the love drain out (don't worry, you're still lovable!).

If you answered mostly 'yes' then I'd like to squeeze your cheeks – stay as lovable as you are!

> 'Every week my partner and I do something really special together. Stuff that's simple and sweet. We take turns who will arrange it.'
> **Anne, 29**

How to love: Try to see the best in your partner no matter what. Be a good listener. Be encouraging and kind. Most of all don't let your ego or pride get in the way; be courageous when it comes to loving people.

How to be loved: Be fallible. Open your heart. Give your most authentic self to the people who love you – they deserve to know the real you. Be generous with your time.

> 'I really have learnt to be a much more patient person. I *know* that I will appreciate my children and I feel so lucky to have what I do. I'm not sure I would have felt this way or quite as passionate about my family if it wasn't for our infertility struggles.' **Eliza, 34**

TTC will make you closer if you …

- keep talking

- don't blame each other if TTC isn't working
- don't dump all your fears and anxieties on each other
- make time together just for fun activities
- stop talking about TTC all the time
- do all the things you used to be interested in as a couple before TTC
- try to make each other's lives easier – especially if you are going through fertility treatment
- be each other's support team
- don't forget to *thank* your partner for everything they do for you
- cry together but laugh together too
- do spontaneous, silly things for each other
- send each other text messages throughout the day
- make each other dinner
- don't make each other worry that just because sex has changed with TTC the passion is 'dead' or the romance is over
- be patient, be kind, keep an open heart.

'TTC jokes are part of our life now. I 'pep talk' his sperm too. It makes us laugh.' **Prue, 35**

'You'll celebrate so much more than the average couple when you do fall pregnant. It was the first time I've ever seen my partner cry.' **Cath, 34**

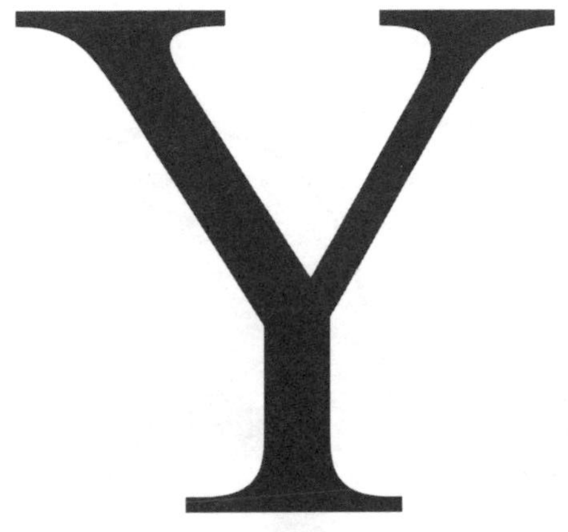

Y is for you

Walking Talking Menstrual Cycle seeks Equally Determined Sperm Dispenser to impregnate her – sooner rather than later. Likes taking temperature, enjoys going for walks to the bathroom and has a good sense of hormones.

That was me when we were TTC and I'm not sure anyone would have answered my personal ad! In between charting,

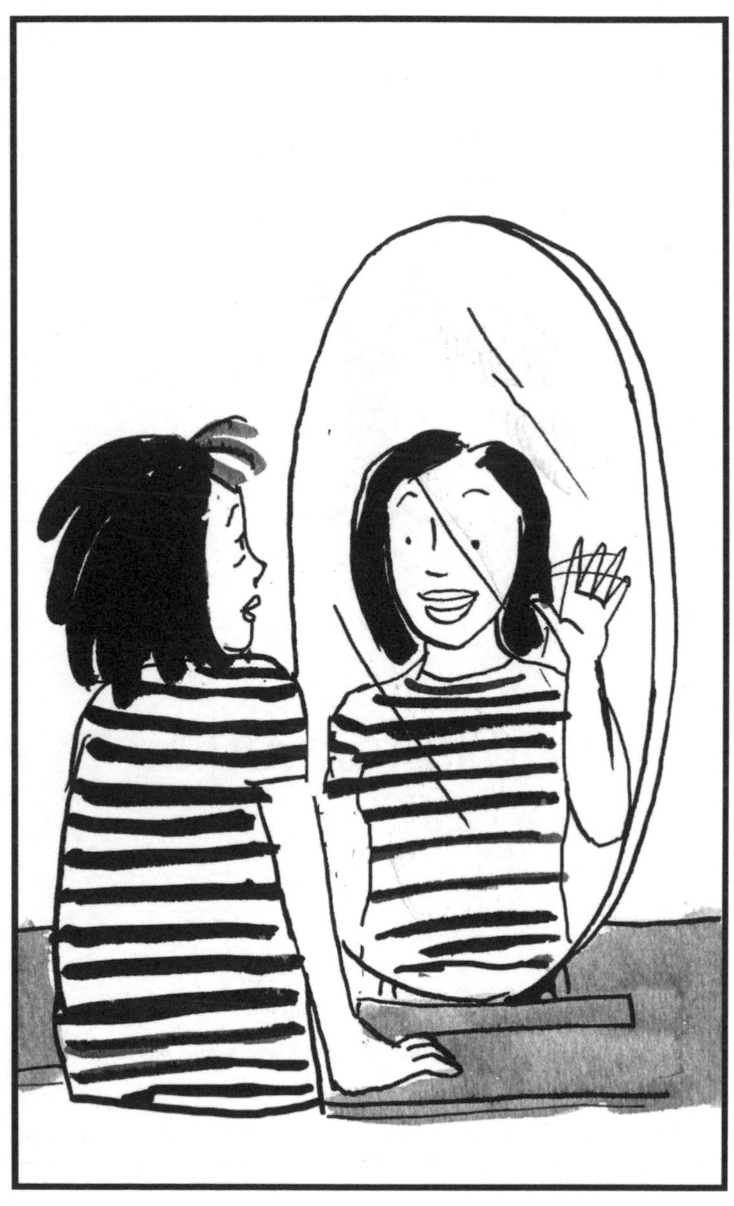

bonking, praying to the Baby Gods and staring at our nipples during the Two Week Wait, it's so easy to lose sight of who we are. Or rather, who we *were* before the baby mission came along. So who were *you*? Here's who I used to be. Genevieve was:

- always planning to go on a detox diet (the planning was more fun than the execution)
- always cuddling and kissing hubby Ben on the couch (before she got grumpy)
- into her job – or at least she used to turn up on time
- trying to get to a pilates class
- organising a weekend breakfast club with her girlfriends
- teaching her puppy Sadie how to sit, stay and not poop in the lounge room.

That was me. So who were *you*? Maybe it's time to give her a call. And this is what you could say: 'Hey *you*. I've been so busy with all this baby-making stuff, I miss *you*!'

And then you could plan a date with you and *you*. It doesn't matter what you do, just do it. Did you use to love shopping, going to the movies, going out for breakfast, or did you love your job?

> 'I took up a course in creative writing and it really helped take my mind off things. I went to the course every Sunday and had to come up with short stories each time – it kept my mind active and on something other than TTC!' **Hannah, 31**

Dates for you and *you*

Don't put your life on hold. Start it again, starting now. Try these you-and-you dates:

- a yoga class
- a long bath with an even longer cocktail (just one!)
- a weekend adult education course
- bungee jumping, sky diving, ice skating (take a girlfriend!)
- that odd little crafty hobby you used to love – remember, knitting is the new *new* yoga
- a long walk on the beach
- a day in the garden
- update your Facebook page
- a trashy magazine to read cover to cover
- a trip to your favourite hardware or garden shop
- a sleep in – *all* morning.

> 'I list all my achievements so far – good job, great husband, fantastic friends. I created that life. That's *me.* That's really something.' **Karen, 38**

The TTC 10-step

But how can I be *me* again when there's so much TTC in my head? On page 269 is the TTC 10-step so you can tear it out, stuff it in your purse or stick it on your fridge to remind you what you need to do every day so you can go back to being *you* and enjoying your life again. This is really all the major stuff you need to know about – unless of course you are undergoing fertility treatment. You can add those must-dos to this list before sticking it to your fridge.

The TTC 10-step

1. Stop worrying, over-thinking or 'bracing yourself' for failure – this is the month!
2. Eat lots of sunflower and pumpkin seeds, oats, eggs, brazil nuts and leafy greens.
3. Have sex like bunnies for at least three days when you see that extra line in an OPK and the LH surge has been detected. When you get to know your cycle, have sex the day *before* you know you'll see that line too.
4. Remind your man to drink his liquid zinc and take a multivitamin every day.
5. 'Refresh' or 'flush out' sperm every three days (all through the month).
6. If you can't improve your cervical mucus – fake it! Try sperm-friendly lubricants such as PreSeed when you know you've ovulating to help the sperm along.
7. Keep warm in the Two Week Wait but remember to chill out!
8. Only have one coffee a day or cut it out completely.
9. Don't have any more than three glasses of wine a week and not in the one sitting.
10. Smile. Remember your affirmations: I am healthy. I am happy. I am a fertile bunny!

'TTC made me feel broken after about a year. I didn't know who I was any more. I was angry and upset all the time. I couldn't be around babies or pregnant women. My life was in slow motion every month as I waited hopelessly to get my period. But it was also racing ahead because I felt like I was running out of time age-wise. I had to mend myself. And that started with working out what I used to love about my life and what made me happy. I was still TTC but I made a point of factoring in those things every day. Silly things like before I was TTC I used to sing in the car on my way to work. I would make myself sing – and *loud*. It made me laugh.' **Helen, 36**

PS: He loves that you, you know. Go get her back!

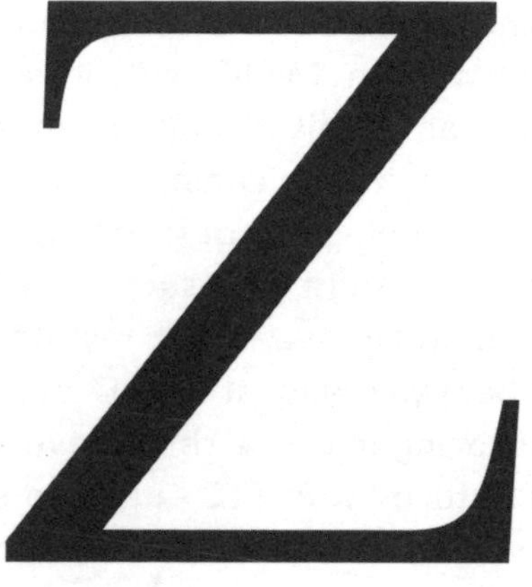

Z is for zzzzz

In between sprogging up and turning up for work on time (even when we get our period) TTC can make you feel as if you haven't had any down time in months. Life gets busy and we often lie awake at night wondering what we can do better next month and when all this TTC is going to end in a pregnancy. But we need our sleep – lots and lots

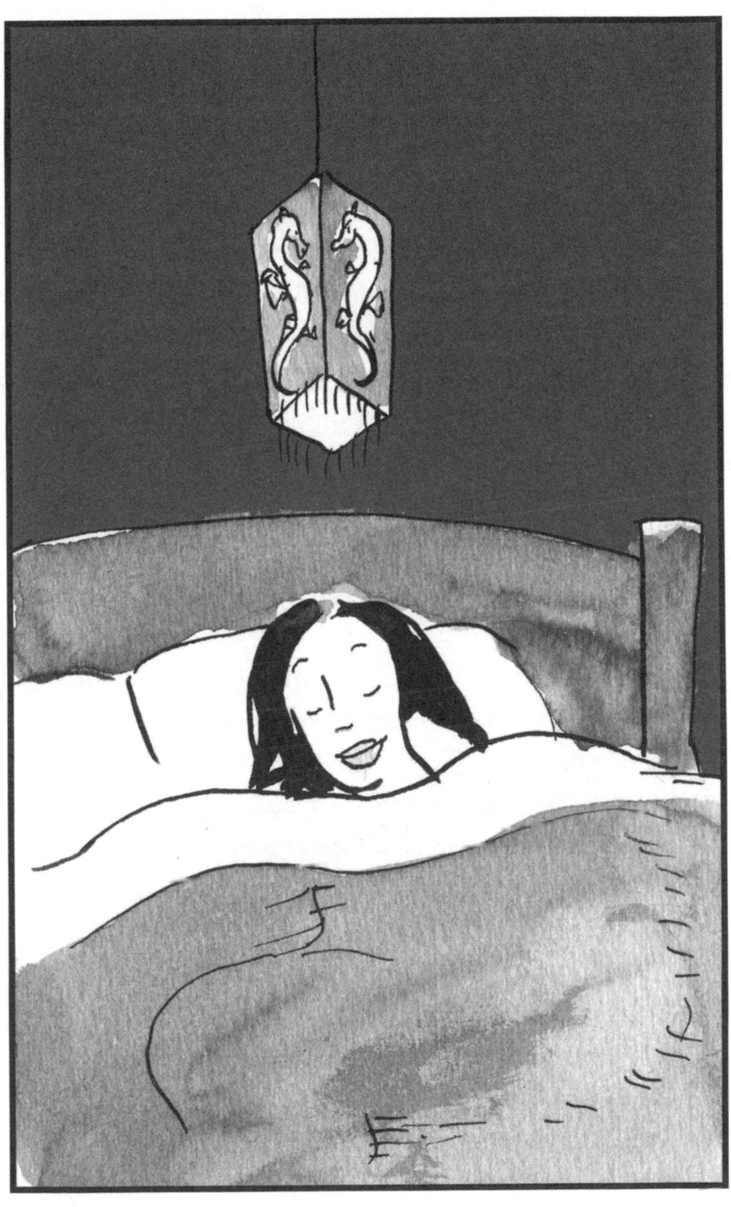

of sleep. Sleep helps restore and rejuvenate the brain and organ systems including the reproductive system. Chinese fertility specialists recommend nine hours a night when you are TTC!

What happens when we don't get enough sleep? When our sleep suffers it affects our mood, our immunity and most importantly, our hormone balance. It can even lead to menstrual irregularity – delaying the time it takes to conceive naturally. Too many sleepless nights can also lead to fertility-unfriendly habits such as too drinking much coffee, comfort eating and unwanted weight gain.

How to sleep better tonight

- Exercise in the morning or in the afternoon – not at night.
- Limit your screen time just before bed, including TV and computers – the flickering stimulates the brain.
- Good sleep-inducing foods include bananas, potatoes, oatmeal and wholemeal bread. Plus the usual suspects like warm milk and chamomile tea.
- Take a nanna nap. Even a 20-minute power nap will do wonders.
- Move to your own bed. If your partner's snoring keeps you awake half the night, find your own bed. You can always crawl back into bed together in the morning.

> 'Fertility specialists in China warn women that without adequate sleep the treatment alone may not do the job. That's how important it is to sleep and to rest. Nine hours sleep a night is recommended when you are TTC.' **Fertility acupuncturist and Chinese herbalist, Shauna Cason**

If you build it, he will come

How sexy is your bedroom? How sleep-friendly is it? The month before Ben and I conceived our baby boy I turned our bedroom into the most tranquil and luscious room in the house. I moved our bed from a room with red walls (red – too much!) and into a lighter room with big windows. I bought a couple of large indoor plants and straight away felt them cool and clean the air. I bought beautiful white cotton sheets and I decorated the room with deliciously smelly candles. Most importantly, I took all my TTC books and newspapers out of the room. I took out anything that was about thinking, worrying, working or planning. From that moment on our bedroom was about love, sex and sleep. So much sleep.

Our bedroom was a happy place. The month we conceived was a really sexy one too. The Fertility Sisters had told us to resist shagging without protection for four months to fully cleanse our bodies and create the best possible egg and sperm for conception (oops) but with all the healthy living, the chilling out and most of all, the relief of finally not worrying so much, we had sex like bunnies for a week.

And I think the sexy bedroom had a lot to do with it!

How to feng shui your bedroom to boost your fertility

This might be silly to some or a solution to others. It might just kill an afternoon during the Two Week Wait. If you've ever wondered what improving the feng shui in your bedroom or your whole house might do for your fertility, from elephants to waterfalls, here's how it's done.

The 7-step fertility feng shui

1. Remove any blocks to the front door. You want a nice open space at the front door as it's considered the 'mouth of chi'.
2. Clean out cluttered closets to allow new, creative fertility-friendly energy to flow more easily.
3. Beds should never share a wall with a kitchen or bathroom. Move it to the other side of the room.
4. Televisions, computers, mirrors and exercise equipment should be removed from the bedroom.
5. Use fertility symbols around the bedroom, including dragons, elephants and double fish (this symbolises double union as in you and your man) and hang red paper lanterns on either side of the bed.
6. Include a mini fountain in your home with clean, circulating water.
7. Plant a fruit tree in your backyard – fruit trees are an ancient symbol of fertility.

Pretty kooky, hey. You're feeling sleepier, sexier and more fertile already!

And just finally ...

Quick Quiz: Will you survive the bump and grind?

1. Have you identified and dodged a Smug Fertility Goddess?
2. Have you sent your family packing for their TTC-insensitive comments?
3. Do you now know what oats and zinc supplements can do for your hubby?
4. Have you made a date with you and *you* yet? And kept it?
5. Do you know now that not having a baby – or another baby – (yet) is not your fault, and that you're not alone and, no matter what, you'll get through the TTC experience?

If you answered mostly 'yes' to the above then you've read this book! If you answered mostly 'no' then make a cup of tea, put your feet up and go back to 'A'.

Just remember, a little bump and grind can be good for you and good fun too! But be very kind to yourself when TTC gets too bumpy and the grind begins to chafe.

And no matter what you do, *do not* relax, not even for a second. *Do not relax!* Stop relaxing immediately. Hey, nobody even say 'relax'!

PS: Everything is going to be okay.

ACKNOWLEDGEMENTS

My most sincere thanks to all in the TTC community who courageously filled out the *Bump & Grind* Questionnaire via email, over the phone and during oh-so-many cups of tea. Thank you for so bravely sharing your TTC stories – grisly bits and all – and for all your support and encouragement during the writing of the book. Thank you to Dr Bill Watkins and Lynne Quayle at TAS IVF and Hobart acupuncturist Shauna Cason for giving your time so graciously. Thank you to The Fertility Sisters for showing me the way (I believe in bunny rabbits!). Thank you to all at Finch Publishing, and especially Samantha, for your warmth and enthusiasm every step of the way. Thank you to the fantastically talented Fiona for illustrating the book and my super-savvy editor Karen. Thank you to my ex-boss, newspaper editor and friend Garry B for never, ever trying to make me a serious news journalist. Thank you to my friends and family and especially to Richard, Annie, Heidi, Natty, Amelda, Georgie and Mazzie for your love and giggles, always.

Thank you, thank you, thank you to my wonderful husband Ben for letting me share our TTC story – semen analysis tests and all! – and for pushing baby Rafferty around the block all bundled up in his pram mid-winter in Tasmania all those mornings when I had to write. Thank you for always believing we'd get there in the end and for your unwavering love and support along the way.

And most of all, thank you to Rafferty, our beautiful baby boy. Thank you for choosing us to be your parents . . . and for inspiring every word.